Radical Remedies

Radical Remedies

AN HERBALIST'S GUIDE TO EMPOWERED SELF-CARE

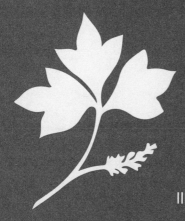

Brittany Ducham

Illustrations by Elana Gabrielle

ROOST BOOKS

CONTENTS

Radical Remedies

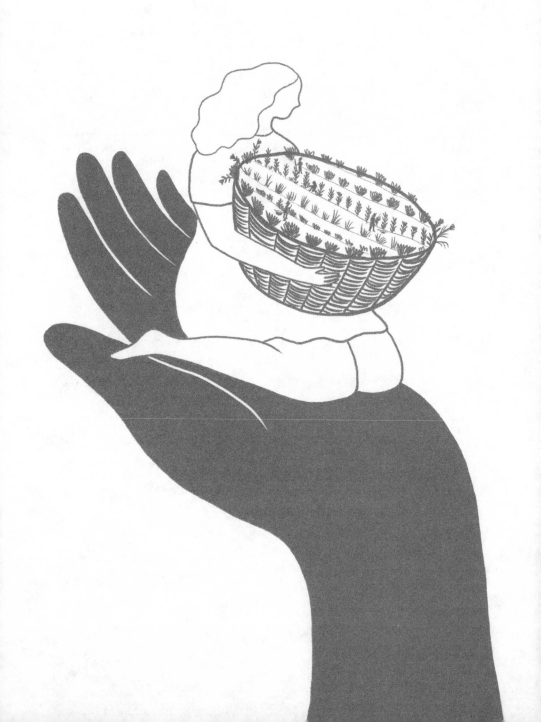

Your Introduction to Empowered Care

PERHAPS YOU'VE HEARD about self-care from your friends or have seen articles about it on the internet. But what is self-care for you? I like to think of it as personalized, everyday habits of well-being—the more we do them, the more we thrive and the healthier we feel. In this way, self-care becomes a lifestyle and an essential way to sustain our personal and collective power long-term.

The good news is that self-care doesn't have to look a certain way or match some type of idealized, presupposed standard. You get to decide what self-care and well-being mean to you based on whatever actions, spiritual practices, foods, people, and medicinal plants make you feel your best. At times, the constant busyness of modern life hinders our ability to tap into the sensitive, adaptive, intelligent, resilient power of the land, plants, and our bodies that our ancestors knew how to harness. The trick to healthy living is to remember—or relearn—that amazing power, to come back to our bodies and heal our relationship with ourselves, and in the process, to reconnect with land and one another so we can all experience care and well-being.

In these times of hyper-productivity, unchecked technology, ecological crisis, and political uncertainty, it becomes crucial to proclaim our fundamental, but often neglected, needs. Basic acts of care can take many forms, from a simple inventory of your most rudimentary needs, such as drinking a big glass of water when you wake up in the morning or preparing a pot of Restorative Overnight Nettle Infusion (page 83) the night before a busy work day, to doing household chores or working on your taxes months in advance. Or, it could be acts that feel more indulgent, imbibing in ritual, pleasure, and rejuvenation such as doing a foot soak (page 208) after a long work day, momentarily hitting pause on your work to walk through the park, pulling tarot cards to better understand an issue in your life, giving yourself a massage with herbal oils (page 214), or investing resources in a local cause that's important to you.

The task of self-care today is to affirm our individual and inherent worth and bridge the new and the old to balance the vitality of our body, the well-being of our societies, and the health of the earth. It can be an overwhelming undertaking, but we are not alone in this work. We have one another and the natural world to learn from and offer support.

Tea or Infusion: What's the Difference?

Water preparations like teas, infusions, and decoctions are tasty and affordable ways to familiarize yourself with medicinal plants and begin building relationships with them. Throughout this book and beyond, you'll notice the terms *tea* and *infusion* are sometimes used interchangeably. What exactly is the difference between herbal teas and herbal infusions? To be honest, not a whole lot. In general, a tea—whether a cup of green, black, or herbal (like chamomile or mint)—requires less plant material and a shorter steep time. When making 1 cup (8 ounces) of herbal tea, use 1 teaspoon of plant material steeped in hot water for 3–10 minutes. Herbal teas are great for a gentle tasting and aromatic brew, which is why herbs like peppermint and chamomile are common.

An herbal infusion requires more plant material and a longer steep time; it is often known as a medicinal-strength infusion (page 221). This preparation is about ingesting herbal medicine and extracting all those water-soluble healing constituents. When making 1 cup (8 ounces) of an herbal infusion, use 1 heaping tablespoon of an herb or herbal blend steeped for a minimum of 10–15 minutes and up to overnight. Herbal infusions taste good, but they have stronger flavors and may take your palate some getting used to. Remember, you can always add honey.

Since water preparations like teas and infusions usually require a bit more time than other herbal preparations, they ask us to reshape our day, setting in motion a different set of healing priorities. In fact, drinking herbal infusions daily is one of my favorite recommendations for anyone who feels run down and unable to relax. Making them is also a great opportunity to practice breathwork (page 109), stare out the window and allow your mind to wander, water your plants, or do some light stretching, all of which help you calm down. Carving out time amid the busyness of your day to prepare and enjoy a cup of tea or an herbal infusion is a powerful proclamation. You are signaling to yourself and others that you are worthy of care and will make time to prioritize yourself so that you feel your best. Even the act of holding a warm mug of tea encourages feelings of warmth and well-being.

Recipes in this book are for medicinal strength herbal infusions as opposed to herbal tea. You're always welcome to use less of a blend and play with different steep times. At the end of the day, what matters most is that you drink your herbs and incorporate them into your practices. Tea or infusion, decoction or broth, tincture or oxymel, you'll find your preference and groove as you go. For more information on hot and cold infusions and decoctions, check out chapter 10, "Your Home Apothecary" (page 219).

That's where this book comes in. We will explore the idea that taking care of ourselves is not a solitary act, that it is through relationships, connections, and empathy with one another and all living beings that true health exists. When we start with simple practices—listening to our body, cultivating emotional intelligence, setting healthy boundaries, exercising, incorporating more whole foods and traditional eating ways, and working with a handful of medicinal plants—we realize that well-being has always been within our reach.

HEALING TOGETHER: A RADICAL ACT

We all benefit from a sense of purpose, the feeling that we matter and that our actions are impacting the greater good. As you take time to care for yourself, remember that your well-being does not exist in a vacuum. Healing together means that for all living beings to thrive we need healthy soil, diverse ecosystems, community, access to affordable housing, nutritious food and health care, clean air and water, and the freedom to be ourselves. As we steward ourselves into health and balance, we must actively do the same for one another and the natural world.

This is reciprocity in action. Reciprocity means we acknowledge that all things are interdependent and require mutual care and tending. All living beings—plants, animals, fungi, people—exist within an elaborate, ever-evolving web. I don't know about you, but when I imagine myself belonging to this web I feel less alone, less disconnected, and more capable of sitting with all that life throws my way.

It is exciting that so many of us are starting to shift how we take ownership of our health. Instead of depending solely on doctors and specialists, we are claiming agency over our own bodies, and even further, we are becoming skilled at growing our own food, using the medicinal plants outside our doors, and advocating for accessible health care in our communities. The act of caring for oneself is not a new activity, though the term *self-care* has emerged as a rallying cry in recent years. As we invest in self-care, we notice the ripple effect, the tides of cultural transformation and community healing that arise as each one of us takes healing into our own hands.

Oftentimes, the race, gender, and class dynamics behind the concept of self-care have gone unspoken. Self-care actually has a rich history, interwoven with social movements and health-care reform, especially in the civil rights, Chicana, and women's rights movements of the late 1960s and 1970s. These movements, which were, and, in many instances, still are led by women of color, help define the role of self-care and illuminate the importance of accessible care options in the face of interlocking forms of oppression. For many, these practices are about basic survival. Financial security, along with access to healthy food, clean water, childcare, affordable housing, well-funded education, and equal pay all factor into how we are able to embark on our self-care journey. Every time we perform an act of self-care, we are honoring the legacy of those who came before us and committing to our fundamental needs, bringing our awareness to the root issue, be it personal or societal.

When we take time to untangle what we have been taught about our worth and decide that we are worthy of prioritizing ourselves, we take a stand for a radical, healthier future. We begin to see that what started as a personal act is innately political, setting a precedent for mutual aid and healing justice for all. When we dare to carve out time for ourselves, dare to imagine and fight for a society that supports the need for personalized and accessible care for all, we let go of what we have been conditioned to believe and reclaim our power.

WHAT PLANTS CAN TEACH US

A reverence for plants, people, and all living organisms is at the core of herbalism and plant medicine. When so much of the world is plagued with struggle and suffering, when the news is full of global warming–induced disasters and mass extinctions, we must take a hard look at whether our current systems are working for humans as well as for all living beings on this planet. It's in times like these that we must be open to regenerative, sustainable, and healing ways of inhabiting our place in the world. Plants and fungi are some of the best teachers for this work. They provide a mirror through which we can better understand ourselves and the world around us. By paying attention to the relationships that plants form with fungi, animals, and one another, we can better understand our lives as interconnected. When we begin to *be with* plants—sitting with them where they are rooted, inviting them into our kitchens, supporting the farmers that tend to them, and asking for their help in moments of stress or crisis—their vast wisdom is revealed. We gain insight into our own natural adaptability, reciprocity, and vulnerability by witnessing these tendencies in the natural world.

To prevent major illnesses and disease, you have to listen to the signals your body is sending you before it finds louder and more harmful symptoms to get your attention. Much of conventional medicine is focused on covering up symptoms until it is too late, but herbs ask us to listen to and respect the body so that we can tend to *both* the symptoms and the root cause. After all, our symptoms are our friends; they are the language by which our body speaks to us. Working with herbs is much more about paying attention to this language day to day and prioritizing prevention, although medicinal plants are versatile, generous, and can continue to support you with their healing capabilities no matter what you're going through.

Integrating medicinal herbs into our healing framework offers an intimacy that is often lost in industrial societies, where doctor's visits often reduce us to our symptoms and biochemical workings, disconnect us from the land, and remove us from growing and preparing our own food and medicine. When we work with herbal medicine, we have a personal, tangible relationship with the plants that guide our healing. We feel connected, empowered, and well. This is why herbalists refer to medicinal plants as herbal allies. Plants are our friends in healing, and it is by building mutually beneficial relationships with them that we can restore our personal and collective health. When dealing with stress, sickness, or disease in the body and in the world, we must call on these herbal allies for guidance and support. Then, with our renewed and fortified well-being, we can show up for one another, defending plants, the land, and all living beings that share this precious moment with us.

ON SUSTAINABILITY AND
ETHICAL HERBALISM

A good rule of thumb as we embark on our personal healing journey is to make sure that the practices, spiritual tools, food we eat, medicinal herbs we purchase, and so on also bring greater healing to the world at large. We should not only question but fight against exploitative industries and mindsets.

Many of us are already accustomed to doing this with the food we eat. We check labels and pay attention to how far our produce has traveled. We advocate for safe working conditions for workers. We shop local as often as we can. You can give the same consideration to how you purchase herbs and herbal medicine. If you live on the East Coast, does it make sense to buy herbs from California? If the herbs were grown in another country, were they picked and processed in an equitable way?

Wildcrafting is the practice of harvesting plants from their wild habitat, typically for the use of food or medicine. Although reconnecting with wild places can be incredibly gratifying, there are many environmental downsides and considerations with regard to wildcrafting, even if such practices are done ethically and with good intentions. Much like the way *natural* has become an ambiguous or even empty term with no set industry standard, *ethical wildcrafting* brings up many unknowns, as you can only guess at what practices are used in the harvesting of a wild plant. This is especially important when considering plants that are endangered or endemic to only one region in the country or world. We are in a state of increasing ecological collapse, so how we, as humans, connect with the land is of life-or-death importance. Take the time to educate yourself, try to grow your own herbs whenever possible, support local and regional growers with trusted practices, and ask questions when anyone claims to use wildcrafted plants.

If a person or store selling wildcrafted plants can't answer any of the following questions, you should not purchase wildcrafted herbs or herbal medicines from them.

→ How much of the plant do you wildcraft at any one time?

→ Do you revisit the same place year after year?

→ How long have you been tending to the same area?

→ How do you steward this area for future generations?

→ Do the indigenous people/tribal communities in your area consent to your harvesting this plant for profit?

→ How do you ensure that the area you're harvesting from is free of contamination and safe?

→ Are you familiar with United Plant Savers and their At-Risk and To-Watch lists?

→ Do you donate a percentage of your sales to support indigenous sovereignty and/or decolonization efforts?

The significance of contemplating wildcrafting practices and your impact on ecosystems is even more important when living in a settler nation. A settler nation is a product of colonization and refers to countries that were settled by Europeans who upon arriving to a place claimed dominion, displacing and erasing—often violently—indigenous populations. Examples include the Americas and Australia. With legacies of colonization and racism still thriving across the globe, you must take a moment to check in with yourself about any assumptions that you are entitled to land and plants. I know this can seem confusing: on one hand, I am encouraging you to have a relationship with medicinal plants, and on the other, I'm insisting that you shouldn't carelessly go into nature and take. As with all things, a balance must be struck. It's key to remember that you can have a relationship with the land and plants without taking them. In fact, there is a growing movement of herbalists who do not wildcraft plants at all. You can walk among, sit with, steward, and grow your own (or financially support the livelihood of someone who does). This is especially true for those of us with European ancestry who have inherited the responsibility to not only heal our current and ancestral wounds but to dismantle oppressive ways of thinking and being that keep others down and consider our earth a source of limitless resources for unchecked human consumption.

A favorite and preferred practice is urban foraging. As a personal rule, I do not wildcraft, but I do spend many hours walking through the neighborhoods where I live and visit getting to know the weeds and naturalized medicinal plants that grow in abundance there. Give it a try! Most of us have common weeds growing in our area, and many of the plants in this book can be found growing in urban settings. Take a look at pages 16–17 for a list of medicinal and edible plants that are common in neighborhoods near you.

The Radical Relationship between Plants and Fungi

As we dive into the wonderful world of medicinal plants, in awe of their ability to heal and teach us, it's worth noting that they aren't the only healers and teachers in the natural world deserving of our respect and admiration. I'm talking about fungi, which are in fact a separate group of intelligent organisms that exist within their own diverse classification system. The plant kingdom comprises trees, flowers, and ferns that derive energy from photosynthesis and the sun. In contrast, the fungal kingdom, which comprises microorganisms like yeasts and molds as well as our beloved medicinal and edible mushrooms, do not photosynthesize and instead break down and absorb nutrients from their surrounding environment.

Reishi and other mushrooms we use for food and medicine are actually only the fruiting body of an elaborate fungal organism that exists below the ground. This underground part is called the *mycelium*, the threadlike, extensive network beneath the soil, much like the neural network of our nervous system. It is through the mycelium that entire ecosystems stay connected and communicate. This mycelium network allows aboveground plants to distribute information and nutrients to one another. That's right: plants, with the assistance of fungi, talk to one another, warning of disease and pests, and signaling changes in soil or air quality. In fact, if a tree in the forest is lacking, nearby trees will redirect their energy and send this tree resources via the fungal mycelium network to help it sustain life.

The world around us is alive and intelligent, and when we create communities that resemble the intricate, reciprocal networks of the fungal and plant world, our lives better come together to enrich the whole.

Some common guidelines for urban foraging are:

→ Keep it simple. Familiarize yourself with dandelion, cleavers, violet, goldenrod, etc., instead of going into the wild and harvesting native species that are already at risk of overharvesting and loss of habitat.

→ Make sure you are 100 percent sure of plant identification. Buy plant ID books and talk with knowledgeable pals, naturalists, or herbalists in your area.

→ Never take more than 10 percent of what you see growing. Just because there is a lot of a plant in your area doesn't mean you should take all of it or make assumptions about its environmental status. Consider the well-being of native pollinators, health of the ecosystem (your neighborhood, town, and/or city is an ecosystem), and future generations of the plant, as well as other responsible nature lovers who might be tending to and enjoying the area.

→ Make sure lawns, parks, etc., where you are picking have not been sprayed with pesticides or otherwise affected by contamination.

→ Ask the plant for permission. This act acknowledges that plants are intelligent and our work with them is about respect for life and relationship building, not careless taking. If a plant never says "no" to you, you aren't actually listening.

A pivotal role for anyone who cares about the earth and its inhabitants is to bring awareness, change, and healing to how we relate to one another, to plants, and to the land by looking critically at how oppression lives in our social, spiritual, and environmental practices.

INTEGRATIVE HEALTH

It's natural to experience a bit of nervousness or intimidation when wanting to work with medicinal herbs. It can feel like a whole new frontier! Our current health culture, referred to as *conventional medicine*, focuses on resolving symptoms of illness with pharmaceutical medication and reduces the body to separate systems with no overlap. For example, many conventional doctors might not see a link between the food you eat and the health of your immune system or acknowledge that your digestive system can impact the health of your nervous system and mood. Within conventional medicine you're likely to go to a specialist who rarely takes a holistic approach to health. This model of health care is slowly starting to become more open to the curative ways of a balanced, plant-based diet, and to the use of medicinal plants and fungi, but there is still a lot of skepticism and doubt. This is actually strange when you consider that almost all pharmaceutical medications are derived from plants and fungi.

Many of us were raised not with plant remedies but instead with an unquestioned confidence in the medical and pharmaceutical systems. This belief is deeply instilled in our cultural understanding of care and can make us unsure of how to work with a different approach. The good news is you don't have to choose one or the other. Prioritizing holistic well-being by utilizing the healing potential of medicinal plants isn't about turning to herbs and forsaking conventional medicine and doctor's visits; instead, it's about acknowledging that by combining and respecting the vast knowledge of many healing systems and approaches we can create and advocate for integrative health care on our own terms.

First and foremost, integrative health emphasizes a holistic, personalized approach to health care and well-being and aims for well-coordinated care between different providers. A fundamental rule for putting together your team of health-care providers is that they should be rooting for you. Don't waste your time and money seeing a health-care practitioner who does not align with your values or support you in getting second opinions or working with practitioners outside of their area of expertise.

PHYSICAL AND ENERGETIC APPROACHES

As you'll learn, there are many ways to think about and work with plants and the natural world. There are also different ways to think about holistic well-being that can set the stage for you to incorporate different herbal preparations and practices into your life.

Some approaches are strictly scientific, backed by research published in journals that are concerned with herbal constituents, chemical processes, and medical understanding. I consider this the realm of physical medicine, where we think mostly in terms of anatomy, physiology, and phenomena we can experience through physical sensations. You're probably already familiar with the dosages and preparations used in physical medicine, as they are the bedrock of conventional medicine and clinical herbalism in the West. Drinking a quart of herbal infusion, taking any kind of prescribed or over-the-counter medication, taking a dropperful or two of tincture, and rubbing a sore muscle salve on your achy neck are all considered physical medicine.

Radical Remedies

United Plant Savers

As you begin learning about herbalism and the medicinal plants growing in your region, take some time to familiarize yourself with United Plant Savers and their At-Risk and To-Watch plant lists. The information shared on these lists can shape how you shop and what medicinal plants you work with. United Plant Savers is a nonprofit organization that works tirelessly to preserve native North American medicinal plants and the ecosystems they call home. Started in the early 1990s by Rosemary Gladstar and other passionate herbalists, United Plant Savers is dedicated to the conservation and cultivation of medicinal plants. Concerned that the growing popularity of herbal medicine, though positive in many ways, could result in the endangerment or even extinction of some of our most beloved medicinal plants, these dedicated herbalists promote reciprocity, education, land stewardship, and responsible consumption.

Other approaches, what I'll call *energetic medicine*, are rooted in many traditional and indigenous healing systems. This variety of medicine is imbibed with spiritual and symbolic meaning, poetic understandings, ancestral remembrance, elemental frameworks, intelligent feeling, and an awareness of subtle energies that go beyond physical sensation. Sometimes referred to as emotional or spiritual medicine, these approaches typically involve smaller dosages and introduce us to different herbal preparations.

Every perspective, whether rooted in the physical realm, the energetic realm, or a combination of both, has a different way of understanding how your emotions can manifest in your body. What's most important to understand is that our emotional and spiritual selves are not separate from the workings of the body. The way you feel has an impact on your life force—and the ability of that force to flow through your body. We can feel this vital energy or spiritual well-being when we're hot with anger but forced to hold it in. We clench up and our skin burns with a feeling of injustice. Emotional build-up can leave us feeling stuck, unbalanced, ashamed, or aimless and can even play into a physical complaint.

In my own practice and within this book, I enjoy a balanced combination of both physical and energetic medicine. I do not believe in forsaking one for the other, as healing happens in many integrative forms and looks different for everyone. You can certainly find a variety of books, practitioners, and teachers that speak to your flavor of herbalism and healing wherever it exists on the spectrum.

WORKING WITH A TRAINED HERBALIST

One of the best things you can do beyond incorporating a few herbs from this book into your routine is to seek out a trained herbal practitioner or herbalist. Look for one with your ideal approach and sit down for an initial consultation to go over your health history and future goals. Nowadays, many trained herbalists offer distance consultation services, so if no one is available in your area, you can usually connect via e-mail, phone, or video chat to get the support and advice you need.

At the end of the day, this book is a jumping-off point and should not be used to replace the one-on-one, personalized insight a trained herbalist can provide. Although everyone can work with and should have access to medicinal herbs and healing knowledge, not everyone is a trained, experienced herbalist. Herbalism is the people's medicine, but that doesn't mean everyone is qualified to be an herbalist and give advice. With herbalism gaining in popularity, many blogs, social media platforms, and editorial websites are publishing herbal information written by a layperson with zero training. These opinion pieces often confuse or water down herbal knowledge, making it difficult for beginners to know what information is credible and trustworthy.

There is no certification board in herbalism, so you have to do your due diligence to find a practitioner who is knowledgeable and qualified. Some trained herbalists may call themselves clinical herbalists, usually meaning they graduated from a school of herbal medicine. There are also folk, energetic, and community herbalists. These practitioners can be equally qualified as clinical herbalists but may have gone the route of self-study and/or learned through an apprenticeship or mentoring program. Often, herbalists have done a combination of all of these, consistently fostering their passion for healing and medicinal plants.

There are many ways to learn about herbal medicine and several ways to categorize herbalists. What matters most is that you find someone who has put in a minimum of four to five years of dedicated study, has experience working with clients, has a relationship with their mentors, and is familiar with your specific condition and needs. Take a moment to consider what exactly you're wanting from an herbalist. This might include someone who:

- → specializes in trauma-informed care
- → has experience with the LGBTQI+ community
- → offers a sliding scale
- → practices energetic herbalism
- → can understand lab results from your general practitioner
- → has experience working with someone already on lots of different medications for varying conditions

If you're interested in working with an herbalist but aren't sure of their background or if they're the right fit, reach out and ask them questions about their training and expertise. If they aren't right for you, it's likely they can recommend someone who is. In addition to the resources (page 241), you can also check out the American Herbalist Guild for a list of practitioners.

SAY YES

In order to fully say yes to our lives, we need to believe we are worthy of care, success, pleasure, love, health, joy, rest, and all the other glorious, life-affirming gifts that we sometimes think we don't deserve. Well, we do—you do! Life is a whole lot better when you say yes to yourself and the path of radical well-being.

Sometimes this work is boring, challenging, and doesn't look pretty—it's about slowing down and giving yourself permission to experience the highs and lows. It's about accountability and reckoning with patterns that hold us back. It's saying yes to yourself, which sometimes means saying no to engaging with people, patterns, and situations that aren't good for you. It's about honoring your intuition, ancestry, and goals for future happiness. Self-care is messy and imperfect, but then again, so is healing. *We* are messy and imperfect. Our capacity for growth is in direct proportion with our willingness to say yes to the dirty, rough-around-the-edges work of healing. Caring for yourself will be a process, an ongoing practice that changes with the seasons, ebbs and flows with your moods (and maybe even the moon), and is always something you can come back to.

This book is meant as an introductory guide to cultivating well-being in modern times—a toolkit full of herbal insights, dietary recommendations, and versatile practices that can support you in moments of stress or hardship as well as infuse your every day with intention and connection. Self-care is a tapestry of personalized actions—big and small—that we enact daily to feel our best and shape the world for the better. The more supportive tools you have, the more empowered you will be. Ultimately, self-care requires us to be brave and to ask ourselves if the very basis of how we live is healthy for ourselves, our families, our country, and the very planet we live on.

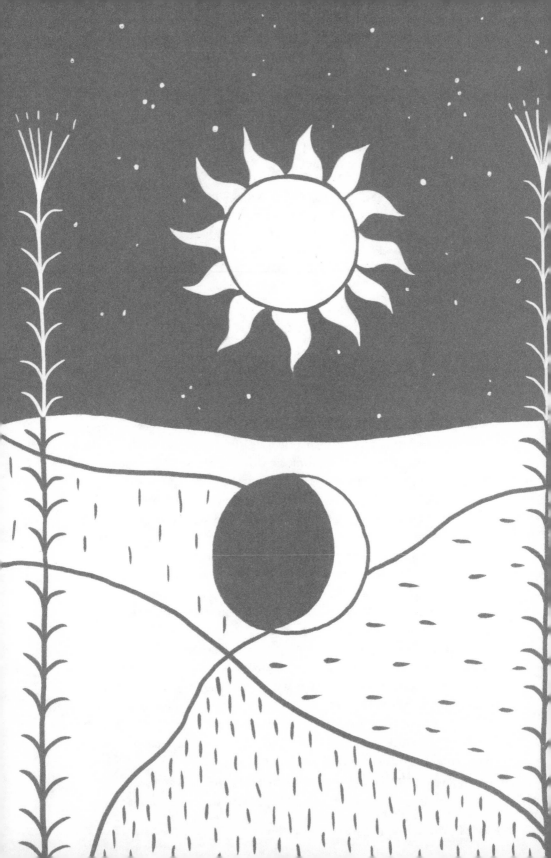

Putting Plant Medicine into Practice

1

HUMAN EXISTENCE HAS BEEN marked by our interdependence with plants. Long before there was the FDA and science as we know it, people have been using plants as food and medicine. The medicinal herbs in this book have been tried and tested through the wisdom of experience and passed on from generation to generation. When we work with herbs, we honor this lineage and awaken something sacred and vital within ourselves.

Herbal medicine is rooted in the belief that plant healing belongs to everyone. Herbal medicine is the *people's* medicine, available to anyone who takes the time to learn about it and thereby take back responsibility for their health. The more you use herbs, the more your body remembers patterns of healthy living. It requires self-awareness and intuition—both necessary tools for all healing paths. This intuition is a subtle knowing that we all have within us, a kind of knowing without knowing, that unexplainable hunch, the gut feeling, the trusted pull of our heart. It's the way many of us come to working with herbs—feeling defeated and frustrated with conventional medicine, we start to trust our own bodies and the idea that there has to be a better way to soothe stress and heal illness.

Your work with herbs can be as varied as the moment requires. You can work with herbal medicine as a tea, a tincture, or an oil; burn an herb for cleansing or protective smoke; sleep with herbs under your pillow; sit with an herb and meditate; take a bath with herbs; rub herbs all over a roast chicken; walk to work and identify herbs as you go; plant them in your garden—the list goes on and on.

STARTING WHERE YOU ARE

When seeking out herbal medicines, whether you want to sit down with a clinical herbalist for a consultation or you're looking to purchase dried or fresh herbs or premade medicines, look to those growers, apothecaries, and medicine makers in your area first. After all, we are shaped by our surroundings. Climate and terrain influence how we experience health, and place is something you have in common with the plants and fungi growing around you. Both you and the plants in your region thrive under specific conditions, and it often ends up that the plants growing right outside your door are the medicines you need the most.

Start in your town or city, with your local farmer's market or plant nursery. Does anyone grow medicinal herbs? Does anyone make herbal medicines? See what turns up. You may be surprised at what you find! Check out the resources (page 241) and at the very least try to support those in your region. This allows you to invest in the people-building sustainable networks of health and healing near you while experiencing a greater connection to the plants and place you call home.

Also, start getting curious about the medicinal herbs right outside your door. Take a walk around your neighborhood, sit in your backyard, or visit a nearby park. Start with the weeds, as you've most likely lived alongside them your entire life, never realizing these powerhouse healers were right under your feet.

Weeds are some of our most abundant and reliable medicines—they teach us how to be resilient, to grow and flourish where we must, and to adapt to our surroundings. It is these humble weeds that remind us to stay simple in our approach to wellness. We can start with the information at hand and the plants growing nearby.

Common weeds and easy-to-forage naturalized plants are:

→ Calendula

→ Catnip, and most mints like peppermint and spearmint

→ Chickweed

→ Cleavers

→ Comfrey

→ Dandelion

→ Elder

→ Evergreens like pine, spruce, juniper

→ Feverfew

→ Garden sage

→ Garlic mustard

→ Goldenrod

→ Hawthorn

→ Lavender

→ Lemon balm

→ Nettle

→ Plantain

- → Rose
- → Rosemary
- → Thyme
- → Violet
- → Yarrow

In particular, the herbs chosen for this book were selected exactly because each one can be used in a multitude of ways, to support various conditions of an individual at different stages of life, and with very few interactions with medications or other negative side effects. These herbs are easy to find, they grow in the United States, and they are commercially available, which makes it easy to keep them on hand.

TRADITIONAL HEALING

Traditional healing is the oldest form of medicine and is rooted in a reverence for the earth. This form of healing relies heavily on medicinal herbs and a nutrient-dense diet that reflects the local landscape. You might think of traditional healing as home remedies lovingly prepared by your grandma, passed down through generations, or the healing systems of Traditional Chinese Medicine or Ayurveda that have been shaped over hundreds or even thousands of years. These examples represent the breadth and diversity of traditional healing, as these approaches to healing reflect the changing needs of every region, religion, and culture across the globe.

Immigration and colonization have spread people and plants across the world, yet these traditions have continued. This has not always been easy, as the suppression and misrepresentation of traditional ways are common tools of colonizing nations. There is great power in being able to heal yourself, in using the resources around you to fortify your health and home, and because of this, traditional knowledge was often threatening to colonizing powers. Historically, women, especially those who lived close to the land, were often the guardians of traditional healing ways, and as the mass consciousness changed as a result of the influence of church and state, these women were labeled witches and outcasts and considered dangerous. We owe a great deal to the wisdom and defiance of traditional healers—wise women, witches, midwives, medicine men, *curanderas*, and shamans—who held fast against harsh new realities that aimed at the violent erasure of traditional peoples and their healing ways, beginning in Europe and subsequently landing on the shores of Africa and the Americas.

Traditional healing systems the world over have similar, underlying themes—which speaks to the effectiveness of these systems. Throughout this book we will rely on some of these principles to frame our contemporary understanding of self-care:

→ Access to healing knowledge is a basic human right.

→ Health and our relationship with our body is an ever-evolving process.

→ Vibrant well-being is the convergence of social, mental, emotional, physical, genetic, environmental, spiritual, and historical influences.

→ Food is medicine, and the health of the digestive system speaks to the health of the whole body.

→ Emotional distress, trauma, and stress can all contribute to disease.

→ There is a universal intelligence that inhabits all things.

→ Herbs, diet, and lifestyle are at the heart of well-being.

→ Symptoms are a sign of a larger systemic imbalance that needs to be addressed in order to heal holistically.

The best way to adopt these principles into your life is by taking cues from the terrain and climate where you live, befriending your body to better understand your individual constitution, supporting regional farmers and medicinal plant growers, and connecting with your own ancestry. Reach out to parents and grandparents to understand the traditional foods and medicines of your personal lineage. If they aren't sure, do some research on your own—we all have indigenous roots somewhere in our lineage, though some of us will have to look back a lot further than others. Research your genealogy and find a book about medicinal plants from your lineage. What plants did your ancestors use to heal? What were their spiritual practices and sacred plants? What was their diet like? Get creative and integrate these ways into your self-care practices, as they create a sense of belonging. After all, traditional healing is about ancestral remembrance and honoring and reviving our personal food and healing traditions. Be conscious of how traditional healing is woven into your personal self-care practices and do your research to avoid appropriating the traditional ways of other cultures.

AN ELEMENTAL APPROACH

Four foundational elements have danced in our psyches since ancient times. There is great healing power when we evoke these sacred forces. When we work with these elements we can meet our specific and ever-changing mental, spiritual, emotional, and physical needs. Fire, air, water, and earth form a classification system that allows us to better understand ourselves, our healing potential, and the best herbal allies for our unique needs.

The elements are a common thread connecting all healing traditions—the five phases of Traditional Chinese Medicine, the three *doshas* of Ayurveda in India, the four directions of Native Americans, and the four humoral temperaments of the ancient Greeks and Arabs that went on to shape Western herbalism and conventional medicine today. Understanding the elements enables us to better understand ourselves and the world around us.

Fire, air, water, and earth are the building blocks for all things: plants, people, the food we eat, and even disease can be categorized by their elemental blueprint. When working with medicinal plants, this blueprint is known as *herbal energetics*. Although the term *energetics* may sound a little out there to some, it is completely scientific and based on sensations and patterns that allow us to classify an herb's unique properties and its effect on a person based on their symptoms. In herbal energetics, the elements take shape in four corresponding qualities. These qualities exist on the spectrum of hot/cold and moist/dry. Note that hot/cold are not based on an actual temperature. For example, aloe is energetically cooling and ginger is energetically warming, though neither of these plants actually have a cool or warm temperature. By using this primal organization system, you give yourself a comprehensive framework to work within. You no longer have to guess which herbs are best. By learning how these elemental qualities manifest, you'll be able to treat both the symptoms and cause of imbalance and support yourself in your personal pursuit of health and well-being.

Everyone contains all four elemental qualities, but typically a person is more dominant on one side of the spectrum. You can be hot/dry, hot/moist, cold/dry, or cold/moist. Again, this doesn't mean that you won't ever experience the other qualities. Rather, you will fluctuate due to external forces like diet, season, weather, illness, or stress, so it's best to think in terms of existing on a shifting spectrum and defining health and balance on your own terms. For example, balance for a person with a generally moist/cool constitution will look different than it would for a person with a dry/cool constitution.

So, these qualities exist in us and in plants. These shared patterns allow us to more accurately pair a particular plant with a person so that personalized healing can occur. If the elements are the building blocks, their qualities are the map, guiding us to better understand the makeup of our individual mind and body. The way these qualities come together creates a distinct internal landscape. This landscape is known as our *constitution*, and by working with our unique constitution we can tap into a more nuanced, individualized form of care.

CLUES TO KNOWING
YOUR CONSTITUTION

The following is a distilled introduction to elemental self-care, though there are many nuances to understanding constitutions and herbal energetics. If you're interested in learning more, seek out a trained practitioner to guide your healing, or look at the resources (page 241) in the back of this book for further reading.

Cold—General tendency toward poor circulation, cold hands and feet, slow digestion, low energy, sluggishness, lack of sensation, difficulty thinking clearly; prefers warm weather; prone to depressed and inactive states of body and mind

Dry—General tendency toward dehydration, scant urine, dry or rough skin, atrophy, overactive mind, nervousness, constipation, decreased adaptability; prefers humid climates

Hot—General tendency toward extroversion, lots of energy, stimulation, face redness, running warm; prone to swollen and inflamed tissues that are hot to the touch, fever, excessive and hyperactive states of body and mind

Moist—General tendency toward runny nose, congestion, mucus, water retention, poor metabolism, oily skin and/or hair, poor immune function; sweats a lot; prefers dry climates

Energetics not only speaks to our physical well-being but also to our emotional and mental tendencies. We've all met people who we consider fiery, outgoing, or quick to anger. We have friends who weep easily or tend to be more empathetic and emotional. These are additional hints that point to a person's constitution. By paying attention, you will quickly realize the underlying elemental workings in your life.

Oftentimes our culture wants one diet, drug, superfood, or herb that fits or fixes everyone. That isn't how health works, though. Although we all have the same parts and may have similar symptoms, our individual constitutions are unique. This explains why my favorite herb for insomnia may not do much for my friend, or how a respiratory herb could actually make someone's cough worse instead of improving it. No two bodies are the same.

Happily, you probably already intuitively understand energetics. At some point you or someone you know has gotten a sunburn or a burn on the kitchen stove. Your first instinct was to comfort the area with cold water, but there are also plants that offer the same cooling relief. When needing to comfort hot, inflamed, burned skin you might grab some aloe or perhaps rose, two herbs that are renowned for cooling and soothing inflamed, hot tissue.

Now let's get a little more complex. Say two people in your life have a cough, but the cough is vastly different in each person. One has a runny nose and a cough with a lot of mucus. The other has a dry cough that makes their lungs feel brittle and on fire. There are many herbs for respiratory conditions and coughs. The most helpful part of an energetic approach is that it narrows down the herbs you will use. Hopping online or grabbing the nearest herb book may leave your head spinning with options, so let's think energetically. You know that the first person has a runny nose, mucus, and is chilled, so they have an excess cold/moist condition and need warming, moving (expectorant) herbs like elecampane, ginger, and thyme. The other has a dry/hot condition, so herbs like licorice, marshmallow root, and rose-hip syrup will offer more relief. So one herb, or one formula, does not fit all, even for seemingly similar symptoms. When we use herbal energetics, we learn ways to more accurately decode our bodies when we are sick or stressed.

Recognizing Energetics

SYMPTOMS OF HEAT	SYMPTOMS OF COLD/COOLING	SYMPTOMS OF MOIST/WET	SYMPTOMS OF DRY
redness	decreased function	mucus/phlegm	loss of function
irritation—physical or mood-related	deficiency	clamminess	decreased adaptability
inflammation	poor circulation	poor immune function	bloating, gas, constipation
swelling	underactive	brain fog	dryness
pain	depression	stagnation	cracking, brittleness
quick to anger	cold hands and feet	water retention	trouble focusing
racing thoughts			anxiety
HELPFUL HERBAL SUGGESTIONS			
burdock root, calendula, chamomile, elder, hawthorn, hibiscus, marshmallow, meadowsweet, motherwort, nettle, oats, passionflower, peach leaf, rose petals and hips, skullcap	ashwagandha, bee balm, catnip, cayenne, damiana, elecampane, fennel, garlic, ginger, gotu kola, holy basil/tulsi, kava, lemon balm, rosemary, thyme, turmeric, valerian	bee balm, burdock, calendula, dandelion root or leaf, echinacea, elderflower and/ or elderberry, elecampane, nettle, pine, plantain, red clover, reishi, sage, thyme, yarrow	ashwagandha, catnip, fennel, gotu kola, holy basil/tulsi, lemon balm, licorice, marshmallow root, oat, seaweeds like nori, skullcap, violet leaf

ELEMENTAL SELF-CARE

When creating a personal self-care routine around the elements, you'll want to factor in both your constitution and any conditions you're dealing with. Cooling herbs and practices balance hot constitutions or conditions and vice versa. Dry constitutions or conditions are balanced by moist, and the opposite is true as well. If you are cold, a cup of tea with warming ginger will do the trick; if you feel flushed, anxious, and irritated, try a tincture of skullcap and passionflower, both cooling herbs for the nervous system.

Generally, you'll work with the condition first while keeping your constitution in mind. For instance, if you tend to be more constitutionally hot/dry year-round you would rely on moistening, cooling, hydrating, and nourishing herbs and foods to balance your constitution day to day. But let's say every fall you get a cold with a runny nose and wet cough, so you would momentarily ease up on all those cooling, moistening remedies and instead reach for warming, stimulating, drying herbs to combat the cough first and foremost. Once the cough is gone you can reassess the energetics that need to be addressed.

TONIC, ACUTE, AND ENERGETIC REMEDIES

A point of overwhelm for many when first learning about herbs is "how do I know which herb to take when?" A simple way to understand and organize the herbs in this book and beyond is based on their use as tonic, acute, or energetic remedies. Often a plant can be all of the above. This might seem confusing, but the simple explanation is that most herbs are suited for many tasks. Like humans, herbs are versatile and rarely do just one thing.

Many medicinal plants contain constituents that can support you in the moment, while consistent dosing over four to six weeks or longer can more drastically shift longstanding issues. The big difference is how regularly you ingest them. For example, let's consider licorice. It's an excellent remedy for sore throats and dry coughs when used as an herbal infusion, syrup, lozenge, or tincture, and therefore is a nice acute remedy when sick. Daily tonic consumption of licorice as an herbal infusion or tincture will showcase its adaptogenic, immune-modulating, adrenal, and nervous-system nourishing qualities. So if you want to work with licorice to gain those adaptogenic qualities, you have to do the work and take it like you would a tonic herb, not an acute herb.

EVERYDAY PREVENTION: TONIC HERBS

A tonic herb is a restorative herb that is taken daily to help tone, build, and balance an organ system or the body as a whole. Tonic herbs are safe and effective when taken in larger quantities daily over long periods of time. A few examples in this book are medicinal mushrooms, adaptogens, and nutritives. These different groups of herbs support vitality, work on deeper imbalances and root causes, and benefit from consistent, daily intake. To build a relationship with a tonic herb and to establish new patterns of health, work with it daily for a minimum of 4–6 weeks.

Tonic herbs require us to prioritize new habits and create lifestyle changes while working with them frequently and continuously. Instead of suppressing symptoms, herbal tonics possess a balancing effect and encourage the body to heal itself. This doesn't mean you won't notice slight shifts in the first few days, or even right after ingesting; it just means that the longer and more consistently you work with these plants, the more you will get out of them.

Taking tonics a couple times a month won't do much to cure your allergies or calm your anxiety. This is when people can get impatient or frustrated with herbs and think they aren't working. We tend to want instant results, and many tonic herbs don't work that way (acute herbs, in the next section, however, do).

Here are some examples of tonic herbs included in this book. The asterisk indicates herbs that can be used interchangeably in both tonic and acute remedies.

→ Ashwagandha (page 84)

→ Calendula (page 72)*

→ Chamomile (page 129)*

→ Damiana (page 159)*

→ Dandelion (page 51)*

→ Elder (page 189)*

→ Feverfew (page 210)*

→ Ginger (page 57)*

→ Gotu kola (page 93)

→ Hawthorn (page 147)*

→ Holy basil/tulsi (page 86)

→ Lemon balm (page 156)*

→ Licorice (page 192)*

→ Marshmallow (page 69)*

→ Motherwort (page 114)*

→ Oatstraw and milky oat (page 103)

→ Passionflower (page 137)*

→ Reishi (page 168)

→ Rose (page 150)*

→ Rosemary (page 90)*

→ Skullcap (page 126)*

→ Stinging Nettle (page 82)

→ St. John's wort (page 216)*

→ Wood betony (page 116)*

	HERBS	SELF-CARE PRACTICES	FOOD NOTES AND HERBAL RECIPES
COOL NEEDS WARMING/ MOVING	ashwagandha damiana elecampane garlic ginger kava rosemary valerian	baths facial steams foot soaks (page 208) self-massage with ginger-infused sesame oil stay cozy in warm socks and blankets vigorous exercise and movement	cook with aromatic herbs eat plenty of broths, soups, and warm foods Ashwagandha Golden Milk (page 85) Banish the Blues Tincture (page 161) Brain-Boosting Infusion (page 95) Breathe Easy Tincture (page 194) Elderberry Chai (page 191) Enliven Elixir (page 160) Sacred Spark Infusion (page 87)
HOT NEEDS COOLING	chamomile cleavers hawthorn marshmallow motherwort passionflower rose skullcap	spray yourself with rose water restorative yoga practice (page 199) less work and more relaxing reaffirm boundaries (page 36) mindfulness meditation avoid inflammatory or otherwise irritating foods like refined sugar, dairy, alcohol, gluten, etc. (page 66)	bitter tastes like dark leafy greens, wild edibles, and salads dark chocolate herbal vinegars; snack on fresh berries, cucumbers, and raw veggies fermented foods like sauerkraut (page 54) Be Cool Iced Tea (page 115) Gut-Healing Infusion (page 73) Hawthorn Rose Honey (page 149) Heart Renewal Tincture (page 148) Inflammation-Soothing Infusion (page 206) Marshmallow Cold Infusion (page 70) Skullcap Bedtime Infusion (page 127) Sustained Calm Infusion (page 139) Tension Tamer Tincture (page 202)

	HERBS	SELF-CARE PRACTICES	FOOD NOTES AND HERBAL RECIPES
DRYING NEEDS HYDRATING/MOISTENING	cinnamon gotu kola holy basil/tulsi licorice marshmallow root oat	thoughtful time with friends intentional alone time stay hydrated with plenty of water drink nutritive-rich herbal infusions oatmeal bath a good book breathwork (page 109) take a fish oil supplement incorporate more healthy fats into diet self-massage with herb-infused oils (page 214)	healthy fats like quality olive oil and ghee whole, cooked foods snack on walnuts and goji berries seaweeds like nori and kelp moistening adaptogens like licorice and ashwagandha Elderberry Chai (page 191) Gotu Kola Rose Facial Oil (page 94) Honey Mallow Soothing Face Mask (page 71) Joy of Missing Out Tincture (page 128) Milky Oat, Ashwagandha, and Rose Tincture (page 104) Nerve Nourish Body Oil (page 217) Trust Your Gut Infusion (page 64)
MOIST NEEDS DRYING/CLEANSING	burdock calendula dandelion elecampane nettle thyme	dry brushing (page 170) body scrubs lighter, smaller meals new hobby invigorating exercise and movement lymphatic massage rituals for release cleanse space by burning rosemary, garden sage, pine, or incense	bitter and astringent flavors cleavers tincture snack on nettle chips elderflower calendula facial steam sautéed dandelion greens Elecampane and Thyme Honey (page 180) Lymph Love Massage Oil (page 173) Roasted Dandelion Coffee Replacement (page 52)

IN A PINCH: ACUTE HERBS

Acute herbs are those to reach for when we need to experience quick results. They are faster acting than tonic herbs, which usually take weeks or months to start improving underlying issues and root causes.

A big difference when working with acute herbs is the frequency by which you take them. With these herbs there's less of a daily regimen and more of a "what do I need in this moment?" approach. So instead of taking a tincture twice a day, morning and night, like you would with your tonic formula, you would take your acute formula only when the complaint occurs and perhaps in much higher doses and more frequently. For example, this might be once a week if you're having trouble getting to sleep on a particular day, once a month for painful periods, or once a year when you get sick with a cold or flu. In these cases, you would take the acute formula hourly, or even every 5–15 minutes, until symptoms subside. This is called *pulse dosing* and is mentioned in the "Anxiety" (page 107) and "Sleeplessness and Insomnia" (page 132) sections in this book. As a general rule, pulse dosing requires you to take 1–4 dropperfuls (30–120 drops). Due to the higher dosage and frequency, I prefer to work with tinctures for acute situations.

If you start to feel feverish, are in the throes of a panic attack, have preflight jitters, or have a hacking cough that's keeping you awake, you want to work with an herb or a blend of herbs that will create noticeable results. Here are some examples of acute herbs in this book. The asterisk indicates herbs that can be used interchangeably in both tonic and acute remedies.

→ Calendula (page 72)*

→ California poppy (page 201)

→ Chamomile (page 129)*

→ Damiana (page 159)*

→ Dandelion (page 51)*

→ Elder (page 189)*

→ Elecampane (page 179)

→ Feverfew (page 210)*

→ Ginger (page 57)*

→ Hawthorn (page 147)*

→ Kava (page 112)

→ Lemon balm (page 156)*

→ Licorice (page 192)*

→ Marshmallow (page 69)*

→ Motherwort (page 114)*

→ Passionflower (page 137)*

→ Rose (page 150)*

→ Rosemary (page 90)*

→ Skullcap (page 126)*

→ St. John's wort (page 216)*

→ Valerian (page 135)

→ Wood betony (page 116)*

EMOTIONAL WELL-BEING: ENERGETIC DOSING

Herbal preparations like flower essences work in such small doses because we are sensitive beings. We have the ability to experience big shifts in health and happiness with only a small nudge from our surroundings. Think of the transformative power of a stranger smiling at you, a sweet note left by a loved one, seeing a favorite plant growing on the side of the road, or even the scientifically proven benefits of placebos—your entire state of mental and emotional well-being can change, creating major physiological shifts. Subtle occurrences can greatly shape our day; the same is true of our health.

One example of an herbal preparation that only requires a small dose, known as a *drop dose*, is a flower essence. Flower essences are particularly fascinating as they are effective, low-dose (only 1–5 drops) botanical preparations that are safe for everyone, including pets and children. For examples of flower essences, look at the Herbs and Flower Essence section in each chapter of this book. They include:

→ Bougainvillea

→ Broom

→ Cotton grass

→ Dandelion

→ Devil's claw

→ Feverfew

→ Jumping cholla

→ Lemon

→ Mimulus

→ Nasturtium

→ Oak

→ Self-heal

→ Wild rose

→ Yarrow

SEASONAL WELLNESS

Living seasonally means learning how to take cues from the natural world. It's about embracing the old ways of those who lived on the land and were guided by the moon, those who created ceremonies to mark the passing of time while integrating modern innovations. With technology and globalization drastically reshaping our lives, offering us immediate access to foods and goods from around the world, we've lost our connection to seasonality, and in so doing we've fallen out of sync. Seasonal living brings us back to our roots. To relearn these skills is to feel more connected with the sacred rhythm of life, to know the distinctive power of summer, autumn, winter, and spring. Being in sync with the seasons goes further than eating what is in season; it encourages us to reflect on how each season alters our mood, energy level, and goals. How can we harness the energy of each season to best accomplish all that we want for ourselves? What's interesting is that our inner rhythms continue to be shaped by the natural world no matter how far removed we may feel. After all, you don't have to be a farmer to live in relationship with natural cycles like the seasons or the moon—you just have to pay attention. At the height of summer when the days are long, we have endless energy; but during the winter months the sun sets early, and we find our energy moving inward and we crave rest. Instead of expecting the same output from ourselves year-round, we can reframe our expectations based on the seasons. After all, in the winter, plants let go of their foliage and go deep into slumber, while animals hibernate. When we recognize how our relationship to health changes throughout the seasons, we can build a support system that allows us to truly thrive.

> More than anything, seasonal wellness is about allowing your environment to inform your habits.

When we expand our awareness beyond our daily experiences and start to think in terms of our monthly and yearly cycles, we will find clues to what self-care practices we need most. The changing seasons can bring out all that we love, but they can also carry upset and harsh weather, conjuring feelings of worthlessness and melancholy. More than anything, seasonal wellness is about allowing your environment to inform your habits. Whether it's the food on your kitchen table, your self-care routine, or any special celebrations or rituals, being attuned to the seasons is about accessing information that may seem hidden or abandoned in our fast-paced, modern times.

Seasonal wellness is an opportunity to refine your self-care practices so they work for your evolving needs. When your self-care is adaptable, when you accept yourself in moments of flux, you give yourself permission to be whole. When we see our inner life reflected in the natural world, we at once feel a sense of reassurance in our body. We feel an inspired sense of belonging and connection to the world around us. To cut oneself off from these teachings is to cut oneself off from the natural way of things.

Work with the chart on pages 30–31 to engage with and support yourself within each distinctive season. Notice the element and energetic qualities each season is defined by. During each season, you may experience an excess of these qualities. By using food, medicinal herbs, and self-care practices, you can bring stability, meaning, and personalized care into each season.

Case Study: Hawthorn

Let's put together all this information with an example. Here is how one plant—in this case, hawthorn (page 147)—can offer different kinds of medicine depending on the dosage and frequency by which it is ingested.

Hawthorn is a plant with a rich history in folklore and healing. The leaves, flowers, and berries of hawthorn can be used in herbal preparations like tinctures, infusions, flower essences, syrups, and more.

Tonic: Hawthorn is renowned for benefiting the cardiovascular and nervous systems and can be used long-term in cases of hypertension, heart attack, cardiovascular disease, and chronic stress.

DOSING: Take twice daily in tincture form and/or drink 1 cup 2–3 times daily as a hot infusion for a minimum of 4–6 weeks.

Acute: Hawthorn is a nice addition in blends to calm stress, soothe anxiety, and bring someone into their body, especially if symptoms manifest in the chest with tightness. It is best paired with other, stronger herbs specific for relaxing the nervous system, like passionflower, motherwort, California poppy, kava, chamomile, and/or skullcap.

DOSING: Take 1–3 dropperfuls of tincture or 1 cup of a hot infusion, taken on the spot, to lessen overwhelm, anxiety, stress, or heartbreak. May need to repeat tincture dosing every 15 minutes to an hour depending on the severity of systems.

Energetic: As a subtle remedy for energetic states, it is exceptional for the emotional heart and encourages healthy boundaries while supporting someone through emotional or spiritual strife like grief, heartbreak, overwhelm, compassion fatigue, and bitterness.

DOSING: Take a drop dose of flower essence or tincture whenever needing encouragement around boundaries, heartbreak, grief, etc.

Winter

ELEMENT
water

ENERGETIC QUALITIES
moist, cold

GUIDING THEMES
rest, reflect, introspection,
nourish, root, seeds of possibility

BE MINDFUL OF
fear, excess eating and drinking,
escapism, stagnation, lethargy,
doom and gloom

**ORGANS/BODY SYSTEMS
TO SUPPORT**
immune, nervous, skin, kidneys

**SUPPORTIVE FOODS
AND HEALING FLAVORS**
hearty, warming soups; fortifying
broth; root vegetables; beans; citrus;
moving, stimulating, aromatic and
pungent herbs and spices

SUPPORTIVE HERBS
ashwagandha, damiana, elder,
ginger, lemon balm, licorice,
mimosa, nettle, oat, reishi,
rosemary, St. John's wort

Spring

ELEMENT
air

ENERGETIC QUALITIES
moist, hot

GUIDING THEMES
movement, creativity,
envision, sprout

BE MINDFUL OF
stress, anger, irritability,
seasonal allergies

**ORGANS/BODY SYSTEMS
TO SUPPORT**
liver, gallbladder, lymph

**SUPPORTIVE FOODS
AND HEALING FLAVORS**
leafy greens, seaweeds like
nori, nourishing foods, bitter
and astringent flavors

SUPPORTIVE HERBS
burdock, chamomile,
chickweed, dandelion leaf,
gotu kola, nettle, violet

Summer

ELEMENT
fire

ENERGETIC QUALITIES
dry, hot

GUIDING THEMES
play, gather, sustain,
expand, bloom

BE MINDFUL OF
lack of focus, overcommitting,
insomnia, worry

**ORGANS/BODY SYSTEMS
TO SUPPORT**
heart, stomach, small intestine

**SUPPORTIVE FOODS
AND HEALING FLAVORS**
fresh fruits and vegetables (such
as berries, cucumbers, tomatoes),
herbal vinegars and oxymels, sour
and bitter flavors

SUPPORTIVE HERBS
calendula, hawthorn, hibiscus,
marshmallow root, motherwort,
passionflower, rose, skullcap

Autumn

ELEMENT
earth

ENERGETIC QUALITIES
dry, cold

GUIDING THEMES
release, ripen, gratitude,
community, vitality, inner fire

BE MINDFUL OF
sadness, grief

**ORGANS/BODY SYSTEMS
TO SUPPORT**
lungs, large intestine

**SUPPORTIVE FOODS
AND HEALING FLAVORS**
pears, apples, cooked vegetables,
garlic, onions, spices (such as
cinnamon, nutmeg, cardamom)

SUPPORTIVE HERBS
elecampane, ginger, holy basil/
tulsi, reishi, rosehips, thyme

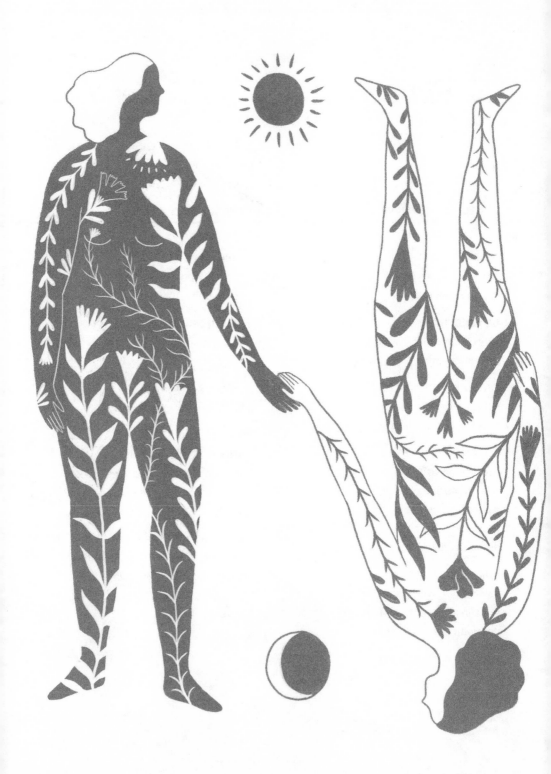

Pillars of
Self-Care

2

WHEN YOU THINK ABOUT IT, taking care of yourself can be pretty straightforward. Get adequate rest, drink plenty of water, eat a balanced, whole-foods diet, and so on. The thing is, we're all so busy juggling our passions, work responsibilities, family commitments, and community engagements that even the most foundational acts often get forgotten or shrugged off.

The pillars of self-care described in this chapter are for you to come back to anytime you feel overwhelmed or off-center. They're the most basic, seemingly unimportant, yet incredibly crucial acts of care. Read and revisit these principles whenever you're going through a stressful time. Write them out on a piece of paper and tape them to your bathroom mirror or the dashboard of your car.

Healthy practices aren't rocket science, but that doesn't mean they'll always be second nature. Trust me, it won't always feel straightforward or easy to stick to these pillars of self-care, but I promise you that in the long run these guidelines will help you show up for yourself and others with more energy and clarity of mind. You'll have more fun and experience rest and calm; you'll feel empowered by your ability to express your emotions and ask for and assert your needs, thereby getting to know yourself in a beautiful, more intimate way.

STAY HYDRATED

Staying hydrated may seem like a no-brainer on our self-care to-do list—after all, we've been hearing that we should drink six to eight cups of water a day since we were kids. Hydration is an essential aspect of optimal health. Maintaining and replenishing fluid levels in the body is vital for muscle and nerve function, joint and brain protection, immune health, digestion, and even mood. Generally, the best way to stay hydrated is to drink enough water and eat plenty of fruits and vegetables, both of which are sources of electrolytes that help regulate fluid levels and hydration. Along with this, we should also consume essential fatty acids commonly found in dark leafy greens, sardines, herring and salmon, walnuts and pine nuts, avocadoes, and by cooking with or drizzling quality olive oil on food.

Electrolytes—sodium, potassium, calcium, magnesium, and phosphate—are minerals that carry an ionic charge that allows the cells, especially the nerves and muscles, to function efficiently. Not only that, electrolytes also play a critical role in how well the kidneys assimilate water for hydration. This is why sports drinks and some bottled-water companies tout their electrolyte content, because as fluids leave the body through sweat or when we are sick, we need to replenish them. Fortunately, there are ways to replenish electrolytes without consuming sugary sports drinks and creating plastic waste. As a matter of fact, most common tap water contains electrolytes, though the amount can vary.

A simple trick to up your electrolytes is to add a pinch of fine-grain sea salt to your water (just enough to subtly taste it, but not enough to feel like you're drinking seawater). Because electrolytes are an essential part of how the cells function, when a pinch of salt is added to water it provides an electrical charge that allows your cells to better conduct energy and communicate with one another. Choose quality sea salt over conventional table salt, which lacks a high mineral content and often contains chemicals and anticaking agents. Himalayan salt is another option, however, be aware that it is being overly mined and is not as sustainable as salt harvested from the sea or rivers.

You can estimate your daily water needs by dividing your body weight in half and drinking that many ounces. Keep it simple by filling up your water bottle or quart jar twice throughout the day. Make an effort to drink 8–16 ounces of water before your morning tea or coffee to start the day off. Caffeinated beverages can be dehydrating, but don't fret, you don't have to give up your coffee or tea habit— just balance it out by drinking plenty of water throughout the day.

ASK FOR SUPPORT

Asking for what you need can sometimes be difficult, as it requires you to be seen, to be vulnerable, and to really believe that you don't have to go it alone. Being vulnerable can be really uncomfortable, but on the other side of that discomfort lies a support system of deeper connection and tools for healing.

When you don't ask for support, you end up alienating yourself from the guidance and resources you need. No one wins when you don't speak up. When you speak up for yourself, you may also be ensuring that others get their needs met as well. After all, we're fundamentally social creatures, and when we're going through something, it helps to be heard and seen and to share the weight of our troubles with others. Support makes us more resilient to all of life's stresses, whether it comes in the form of the insight of a trusted friend or a community support group; as strategies suggested by an unbiased professional counselor, health-care provider, or trained herbalist; the caring touch of a massage therapist; or even a simple heartfelt hug. There is no shame in recognizing that something you're going through is bigger than yourself alone. All you have to do is give yourself permission to ask for what you need.

Sometimes, even when we have the support of loved ones, we have to take responsibility for our healing and seek added professional help. Who doesn't need extra insight on how to understand their thoughts, moods, and behavior? Getting help from a counselor or therapist or some other trained health-care provider can better equip you to dissect a problem and then solve it. This kind of weekly or monthly support can be financially difficult for some people, so look for healers and therapists who offer a sliding-scale option or who do pro bono (free) work with clients with limited income (check out the resources, page 241). Alternatively, get a library card and read self-help books from authors who inspire you, or look into what kinds of support groups your community offers.

> When you don't ask for support, you end up alienating yourself from the guidance and resources you need. No one wins when you don't speak up.

Make a commitment to prioritize your resources so you can sit down with a therapist, trained herbalist, or alternative healer when need be. Do your best to provide a nurturing network of care for yourself and ask for what you need, recognizing that part of self-care means surrounding yourself with people who are on your side, because you deserve to be supported.

SETTING BOUNDARIES

We all need effective personal boundaries that act as guidelines for how others treat us, that speak to our need for balance in life and work and determine how much of the external world we let in. Boundaries are crucial if you work with others in a caregiving, teaching, or healing role, as you can easily get bogged down with what others are going through. And if you're the person in your family or group of friends whom everyone comes to for advice and support, boundaries determine how much energy you give out and what you let in.

In essence, having solid boundaries is about what you say yes or no to; boundaries are about where you end and others begin, about what's okay and what's not. They define who you are in relation to others and should be clear, firm but flexible, and properly communicated. We might get mad at someone for taking advantage of our time or distracting us from an important project, but at the end of the day we must be responsible for letting people know what our boundaries are and sticking to them. This starts with self-awareness and learning to advocate for your needs. Setting boundaries isn't selfish; it's recognizing that to give yourself fully to people and activities that are meaningful to you, you have to use your energy wisely. We can't do it all, and trying to be everything for everyone is a surefire way to experience burnout.

When boundaries are loose, you may easily take on the emotions and needs of others. Common signs of loose boundaries include overinvolvement in others' lives, people-pleasing, trying to fix and control others with judgments and advice, staying in unhealthy relationships, or taking on too much work or too many commitments. When your boundaries are too loose, you can feel responsible for everything and everyone, powerless, imposed on, and resentful.

Pay attention to the people who drain you and the people who energize you. On a piece of paper, list some instances when you have felt emotionally or mentally drained or like your time, personal space, or needs weren't respected. If you can't remove yourself from those situations completely, work with hawthorn or yarrow flower essence.

Anytime you start to feel overwhelmed about the feelings, needs, energies, or "vibes" of others, take a few drops of flower essence, take a deep breath, and find your center. If someone is waiting for an answer or demands your time, let them know you need a few moments and will get back to them. You can say you will get back to them soon, that you need to check your calendar, or excuse yourself in some other way if you don't want to let them know you need to step away to breathe and find your boundaries.

GET REST

Sometimes it seems like everyone is tired. Our most common complaints are fatigue, insomnia, anxiety, apathy, and overwhelm, so it's not surprising that rest isn't as prized as it should be. Then again, when a society considers productivity and an overly full life to be virtuous, it's no wonder we all experience burnout. Instead of resting, we drink coffee or energy drinks, or we misunderstand and therefore misuse adaptogens like ginseng or ashwagandha in an attempt to fuel our busy lifestyles, when what we really need, mentally and physically, is relaxation and repose.

Many of us consider rest the ultimate luxury, but rest is about much more than a good night's sleep or an expensive weekend getaway. It's about combatting the feeling of urgency to do that keeps us from being present and content. It's about releasing ourselves from the notion that our worth is measured in doing as much as possible instead of simply being. We don't have to cross off everything on our to-do lists to earn rest and consider ourselves a good person.

More than anything, you have to let go of the idea that you have to constantly be working to be worthy or successful. In fact, rest, reflection, and relaxation are essential to accomplishing everything you want to accomplish. Build a life for yourself that allows for rejuvenating activities, whatever that means to you. For some that's a quiet night soaking in a bath, for others it's enjoying live music or hanging out with friends. Not everyone recharges in the same way; all that matters is that we prioritize time to do it.

One straightforward way to get more rest and experience more presence day-to-day is to detach from your phone, even if just for a few moments. Try putting down your phone or computer for 15–30 minutes to allow your brain to quiet. Let yourself stare off into space. Focus on your breath. Daydream. You'll be amazed at how wired and exhausted your brain is simply because most of us never actually give it time to turn off. Many of us even sleep with our phones next to our heads—it's often the first and last thing we look at, and that distracts us from fully sinking into the rest we need. Try charging your phone overnight outside of your bedroom and give yourself a break.

OPEN YOURSELF TO JOY

We all have our own reasons why we don't seek out more pleasure and joy. We don't think we deserve to, we feel guilty, we're too busy with work or other commitments, we haven't been shown healthy models of seeking out joy and pleasure, and so on. But on a fundamental level, we need joy to maintain good health. Pleasure and joy are radical, essential tasks for a life fully lived.

Orienting ourselves so that each day we rise with a sense of possibility and curiosity about how and when joy will greet us takes a little effort, of course. Many of us were not taught that fun, joy, laughter, and pleasure are inherent to life. In fact, most of us were probably taught the complete opposite. Let me be clear—life isn't always going to be fun and effortless, but even in difficult moments we can find reasons to live and be grateful. We can invite joy in and seek out pleasure. Not only can we, but we should! Togetherness and creativity are often keys to joy and pleasure, so consider acts that incorporate one or both. Much like how depression and anxiety take a physiological toll, depleting and affecting our entire body and putting us at risk for a whole host of health issues, experiencing joy and pleasure does the opposite.

List-making is a great tool when you need to create an action plan, reflect on situations or experiences, or bring a bunch of fuzzy, unclear ideas, thoughts, and feelings down to earth. This is a riff on a gratitude list, though the emphasis is on encouraging yourself to focus on and follow the pleasurable, joyful things in life. Think of all the experiences and activities you do in a given week or month that bring you joy and pleasure and write them down. Consider how often you feel completely and positively absorbed in a task, those activities that make time irrelevant, that allow you to feel free, relaxed, ecstatic, and present. If you have a long list, if your life is full of daily or weekly moments of joy, relaxation, and pleasure, take time to be grateful and continue to prioritize those things. Work with a tincture of damiana, rose, and reishi to fortify your joyful spirit and continue to steer yourself toward pleasure in all its forms.

On the other hand, if you're sitting there wondering how on earth you've gone so long without feeling a deep sense of pleasure in your life, or if you can't remember when you last had a deep belly laugh, felt giddy with anticipation, or lost yourself in something you enjoyed, your list may take a different form. Write down the things you want to try, sit and reflect on the moments and activities that brought joy into your life at one point, going as far back as childhood if necessary, and consider how you can welcome those experiences back into your life. Work with an herbal infusion of rose, holy basil/tulsi, and fresh ginger to ignite your inner fire, open yourself up to new experiences, and strengthen your conviction for joy.

Radical Remedies

BE ACCOUNTABLE

Personal accountability plays a big role in self-care, because taking care of yourself is largely self-motivated work. Along the way you'll have support and encouragement, but no one can force you to take care of yourself. It's one thing to want to invest in self-care practices; it's quite another to actually do self-care daily, weekly, and monthly.

You get to decide whether you're going to take care of yourself or not. *You* get to prioritize your practices, hold yourself accountable for what you say and do, cook healthy meals, make herbal infusions, be honest about your needs, get out of bed and drink a glass of water, give yourself time to rest, address and set boundaries that remove toxic people and situations, and determine what your time and energy should go toward. And when you fall out of step with what's best for you, hold yourself accountable and renew your pledge to take care of yourself, and don't allow harmful self-talk to take over with negative messages.

Especially during times of struggle and stress, staying accountable to yourself matters the most. Healing isn't linear, and being accountable to your own healing process requires patience and dedication. We're going to have setbacks. We're going to feel deflated and uncertain, depressed, and frustrated. We're going to repeat unhealthy patterns and experience heartbreak. We'll feel like we're doing everything right, moving forward in life, only to be knocked back. This is the time to ask for support and say yes to the care we need while maintaining a level of commitment to our health and healing.

It can feel like extra work some days, but when you commit to self-care you have to commit to showing up on your own behalf. That can be hard work. This is when an accountability check-in can be extremely useful. Create a support system with your loved ones so everyone can feel supported in their journey for mental, emotional, physical, and spiritual well-being.

> Healing isn't linear, and being accountable to your
> own healing process requires patience and dedication.

These check-ins can be self-regulated, or you can ask your partner, friend, co-worker, family member, or therapist to help you stay on track. Consider making your technology work for you by having your phone send you morning reminders that say "Take tincture! You deserve to feel your best," or "Step outside and take a deep breath" when you usually take your lunch break sitting at your desk, or "Drink water," because we all forget to do that.

MOVE YOUR BODY

Having a movement practice can look like having an exercise routine, but it doesn't have to be limited to a typical fitness activity. It really just means that you're intentionally working with your body to use movement to shift mental and emotional energy, reduce stress, and encourage bodily appreciation. Movement builds strength and stamina, and when combined with focus and conscious breathing, it brings us into our being, clears the mind, boosts energy and self-esteem, and keeps our internal systems working. When we recognize that movement has such profound effects, we can create a practice that is as adaptable and therapeutic as we need it to be. It doesn't have to be complicated or strenuous, it only has to help us feel good.

For some, a movement practice is an invigorating evening run after a tough day at work, an empowering kickboxing class, time spent weeding the yard, the spiritual centering of yoga or bowing in prayer, or a weekend hike or canoe trip. Gardening is a movement practice; so is having sex, walking your dog, rock climbing, tai chi, swimming laps, riding a bike, dancing, climbing a tree, or just bending forward and touching your toes. Group sports like soccer, baseball, volleyball, or bowling can get you moving, breathing, and releasing negativity.

Whether your preference is movement that is gentle or vigorous, solitary or with a group, is totally your choice. Shake off any pressure to have a certain kind of exercise routine or movement practice. Movement should be fun and freeing. Depending on who you are and what your needs are, your movement practice can and should vary. Do something that works for you, no matter your age, ability, or state of mind.

BE EMOTIONAL

Supporting your emotions is crucial to holistic self-care. Oftentimes we experience a sense of skepticism around our emotions. We've been taught not to trust them or to ignore or suppress them. We live in a society that is very uncomfortable with emotional openness, and it's rare that people open up about their mental and emotional well-being. When we do see emotions expressed in media, they are often mean-spirited, aggressive, and reactionary. Because of this, many of us were never taught or rarely experience how to effectively communicate our emotions, and consequently we often struggle over how to speak up and advocate for our needs.

When we suppress our emotions, we can inadvertently pick up unhealthy ways of emotional expression, such as avoidance habits like self-medicating with drinking, drugs, food, shopping, or escaping into television or the lives of others. This escapism creates greater disconnection from our authentic selves, and at its worst it pushes away those we hold dear.

Noticing the way we feel emotionally is incredibly useful information worthy of our heartfelt attention and tenderness. By developing emotionally supportive practices, we can constructively channel our emotions. We let our emotions teach us, but not control us. We sit with our emotions, reacting less and listening more. We learn that not every feeling is final or forever. In fact, times of emotional hardship can be the birthplace of spiritual transformation, collective action, deeper intimacy, and creativity. With the support of herbs and other therapeutic tools like a movement practice, quiet time to process emotions, mindfulness meditation, journaling, community support, and therapy, we can begin to appreciate and understand how we feel in any given moment and become more emotionally literate.

One of my favorite practices for emotional processing and release combines ritual and journaling. You begin by asking yourself, "What emotion or pattern am I holding on to that no longer serves me?" or "How can I channel this emotion in a renewed way that benefits me or the greater good?" Once you have identified which emotion or pattern you want to release, take some time to journal about working through and releasing this emotion. This practice is about releasing the hold an emotion has on you so you aren't as reactionary and can begin to create some distance and understanding within that particular situation, pattern, or feeling. You are bringing awareness into how you let the emotion affect you. Letting go, especially of larger emotional upsets, takes considerable time and cannot be rushed, no matter how painful or uncomfortable, and in some cases the wounds never fully heal. In these times, we might work to release counterproductive things like comparing, self-hatred, impatience, and shame, which tell us we should quickly get over life's hardships and keep moving.

A nice way to incorporate plants into this is to burn dried herbs like garden sage, rosemary, pine, or your favorite incense. After journaling, open up some windows and walk through your space with the incense stick or herbs. Let the smoke cleanse the space and reset the room. A great time to do this type of work is during the new moon, as traditionally this is a time of new beginnings and a fresh start.

ACCEPT YOURSELF

Being in our bodies isn't always easy, and for those of us who don't fit society's narrow notions of acceptable—whether based on our appearance, gender, race, size, self-expression, or capabilities—self-acceptance can be even more of a struggle. Liking ourselves, treating ourselves like we would treat a good friend, is a consistent practice we can always come back to.

Oftentimes we think we know how our life *should* be. This could include the kinds of friends we think we should have, the trajectory our career path or education should take, our diet and appearance, the kind of romantic relationships we should have, even our self-care practices. Sometimes society's expectations or our own ideas about what our life should be don't hold up to the reality of who we are and what our bodies need to flourish. Instead of fighting against your nature, focus on the things you can accept and embrace who you are. This can be an incredibly radical act, especially when we don't feel validated and loved by the world around us. Do this by investing in practices that support you.

One way to strengthen this idea is with positive self-talk. Studies show that affirmations and self-acceptance practices help with problem-solving and creativity when we're overly stressed. An affirmation is a conscious thought that you repeat to yourself. This thought is positive and powerful and aims to support you in some way. When we're under stress, we tend to fall back on old scripts. Affirmations train your brain to create a script that promotes a healthy self-image. As we make affirmations work for us, we can translate those healthy thoughts into words and eventually into healthy actions that build the kind of life we want to live.

Positive self-talk is vital to health and long-term healing. The way we talk to ourselves matters. Take some time today, this week, this month, to notice the inner dialogue you have with yourself. If you don't know what I mean, just wait until you're having a particularly hard day and observe your thoughts. We all have certain areas in life that bring up self-defeating stories about what we're capable of. The truth is, being kind, accepting, and compassionate with oneself is some of the hardest work of self-care.

Affirming our healthy habits helps us stay committed when breaking out of old patterns. Instead of focusing on everything we can't do, we affirm the positive, healthy choices we can make. Deliberate, positive self-talk combined with proactive actions build long-term healing. Creating an affirmation practice has the potential to shift your confidence and self-esteem. Affirmations are a great way to tap into your strengths, focus on the good in your life, uplift your mood, and create a more positive reality in the present.

Most of my favorite affirmations are short and simple phrases that are easy to repeat to myself, scribble in my journal, or pin to my mirror:

→ I am enough.

→ Let it be easy.

→ I trust my creative vision and the power of what I have to offer.

→ I radiate love and the universe reflects love back.

→ I am of service to something greater than myself.

→ *No* is a full sentence.

→ I am successful and attract abundance.

→ I am safe and comfortable in my body.

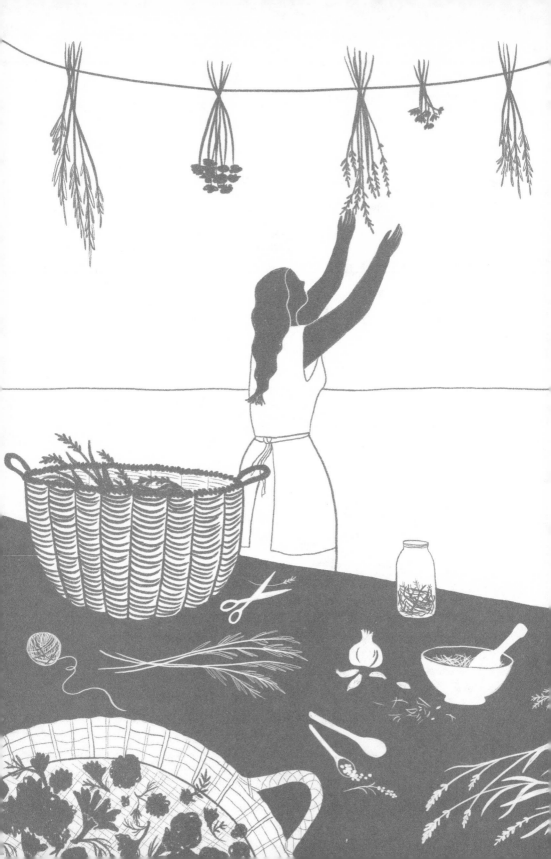

Digestion as the Foundation of Health

3

THE GASTROINTESTINAL TRACT, or gut, is amazingly complex. We're hearing more and more about the importance of a well-functioning gut and beneficial gut flora when it comes to health and happiness. From its impact on everything from mood to immunity, the gastrointestinal tract and digestive system as a whole plays a critical part in our overall well-being. But what exactly is it? Anatomically speaking, the gastrointestinal tract, or gut, is composed of the mouth, esophagus, stomach, and small and large intestines. When we think about the digestive system as a whole, we include the liver, pancreas, and gallbladder. At a glance, a healthy digestive system is the gut working together with the liver, pancreas, and gallbladder to orchestrate the breakdown of food, absorption of nutrients, and removal of waste, but that's not all.

The gut is often referred to as the "second brain," as it is the only organ to boast its own independent nervous system. This system, known as the enteric nervous system, is an intricate network of 100 million neurons embedded in the gut wall. In many ways, we're still learning to what extent the gut and enteric nervous system affect our mood and overall state of mind. Although the enteric nervous system doesn't relay thoughts, it does speak to us in the form of gut sensations and is constantly in communication with the brain. The enteric nervous system makes use of more than thirty neurotransmitters such as dopamine and serotonin, most of which are identical to the ones found in the central nervous system. In fact, more than 90 percent of the body's serotonin lies in the digestive tract, as well as about

50 percent of the body's dopamine. These neurotransmitters play a huge role in our ability to feel happy and experience states of calm. Dopamine is responsible for feelings related to love, joy, pleasure, reward, and motivation. Serotonin helps regulate mood, irritability, impulse, obsession, and memory.

Diet, good digestion, and mood are incredibly linked yet often completely overlooked. An inflamed or otherwise troubled gut can send signals to the brain that causes disturbances in how we think and feel. Issues like brain fog, forgetfulness, irritability, anxiety, depression, and fatigue could be signals that your gut needs some extra TLC.

Whole Foods, Whole Plants

Just as we want to incorporate as many whole, nutrient-dense foods as possible into our diet, we also want to work with whole medicinal plants whenever we can. The great thing about working with whole plants instead of isolated constituents is that whole plants support and balance our entire being, versus acting on one system or mechanism in the body. We often pigeonhole herbs with singular uses when really most medicinal herbs carry an affinity for many different systems in the body. Herbs that promote healthy digestion have a host of uses in the body. Not only do they aid in the digestive process, these herbs have the potential to soothe systemic inflammation, strengthen the nervous system, provide essential vitamins and minerals, and improve circulation, lymph movement, cardiovascular health, mental clarity and focus, and so much more.

In addition, you'll find there's plenty of crossover between your home apothecary and kitchen essentials. In fact, many medicinal herbs may already be in your spice cabinet. By cooking with them more often and using them in the recipes in this book, you'll open yourself to vast healing potentials as well as improved digestion and overall gut health without having to spend a penny on herbal supplements.

Optimizing Your Diet

Much of the illness in the country, digestive or otherwise, can be traced to diet and poor nutrition. If you're lucky, parents or grandparents passed down beloved recipes and taught you the basics of using herbs and spices while cooking and preparing delicious meals. Increasingly, though, this is not the case. Our food system today is vastly different than what our relatives experienced a few generations ago. In the process, we've lost the joy and purpose inherent in growing our own food, along with the wisdom of how to preserve and prepare it. We gained a food system that promises efficiency and ease but isn't overly concerned with promoting health—ours or the health of the soil, water, plants, animals, and workers that we depend on. By working to create meals and self-care practices that combine a whole-foods, nutrient-dense diet with both fresh and dried herbs and spices, we begin to bridge the gap between our modern lives and the healing food ways that came before.

The foundation of health is a balanced diet and well-functioning digestive system. The truth is, no herb, supplement, medication, or surgery is going to negate the importance of a quality diet and healthy relationship with food. Take some time to consider which diet choices are serving you and which are keeping you in an unhealthy cycle. It doesn't have to be complicated. To start, eat more fresh fruits and vegetables daily. Learn to cook vegetables so they taste good and are enjoyable. Take a cooking class, watch YouTube how-to videos, and visit recipe and food blogs that highlight healthy meals and make cooking feel approachable and simple.

LIFESTYLE

Well-functioning digestion is as much about the diversity and quality of food we put in our bodies as it is about how efficiently our digestive system works. Issues can arise in the upper GI (mouth, pharynx, esophagus, stomach, and duodenum) due to stress, not chewing food sufficiently, imbalance of stomach acid, lack of tone in stomach muscles that assist in the breakdown of food, or a poorly functioning sphincter that allows stomach acid to get into the esophagus, resulting in heartburn and gastroesophageal reflux disease (GERD),

Issues in the lower GI (small and large intestines) can arise from eating diets that are low in fiber, not getting enough exercise, experiencing stress or changes in routine, eating large amounts of processed and refined foods and/or inflammatory foods that you may be sensitive to (sugar, alcohol, caffeine, gluten, dairy, soy), resisting the urge to have a bowel movement, and taking certain medications.

PRACTICE: BE A KITCHEN WITCH

The foundation of your digestive power is in how you take care of and feed yourself. For centuries the work and care that went into home-cooked meals was undervalued, mostly due to sexism. Working with medicinal plants has been more or less on the fringes of society, which is always where you find the witch. To honor the overlooked women's work that came before you and tap into the wisdom of the witch you must first reclaim the kitchen as a sacred space filled with magical healing potential. Here are some easy ways you can begin to ignite magic, foster health, honor the old ways, and channel your inner witch.

→ **Drink herbal infusions:** Whether it's a store-bought tea bag, a handful of herbs gathered from your garden or on a neighborhood walk, or a blend you've crafted from the herbs in this book, take time to enjoy tea daily.

→ **Play with your food:** Experiment with new recipes and ingredients, different cooking techniques, and herbs and spices. Incorporate your favorite medicinal herbs into your meals. Check out different markets that highlight culinary traditions you aren't familiar with or are part of your ancestral lineage. Most importantly, focus on fun and play, not perfectionism or getting the recipe just right on the first try.

→ **Cooking is healing time:** It isn't only about eating the meals we make and ingesting the herbal preparations we craft. The intention that goes into the cooking process itself is where the magic lies. The energy you instill into your meals and medicines matters, so respect your kitchen as a special space.

→ **Weekly food prep:** Spend a day or two a week working in the kitchen doing meal prep. Make broth, wash and chop all your vegetables for the week, soak grains and beans for easier digestions, etc.

→ **Find insight and inspiration from the food traditions of your great-great-grandparents:** Buy a cookbook from a country or region that you have ancestral ties to, ask your parents if they have saved recipes or favorite meals that their grandparents made. Take the time to do more from scratch (now that you have a designated prep day), experiment with fermentation, buy dried beans instead of canned and soak them, and so on.

→ **Think sustainably:** Buy ingredients and kitchen tools that are ethically sourced and good not only for your own body but also for others and the earth. Everything we use or consume comes from somewhere. What are the environmental and humanitarian implications of your kitchen staples? How can you limit your plastic?

→ **Share your food:** Host friends and family, or organize a monthly dinner club or potluck. Healing comes in many forms, and community certainly is one of them.

Food Prep: Keep It Simple

Healthy eating is oftentimes about getting back to basics. Ask yourself what foods or meals do you already eat in a given week that make you feel the most sustained and nourished? Now cook those foods more often. You don't need to reinvent the wheel or cook multiple courses to experience the physical, spiritual, mental, and emotional benefits of making food and medicine in your kitchen. It's amazing what putting thought, time, and energy into simple food planning and preparation can do for your overall well-being.

One day a week, set aside time to prep some nutritious snacks and meals for the week. Then instead of ending the day exhausted by the idea of cooking dinner or skipping breakfast because you woke up late, you will already have the basics prepped for a healthy and easy meal. If you're like me and tend to have a hard time coming up with elaborate recipes or don't have the energy to make something healthy for yourself, meal-prepping can be a lifesaver. This can be especially helpful if you live alone and often feel unmotivated to cook for one.

Roast a week's worth of vegetables, steam dark leafy greens, cook a large pot of rice and beans, cut berries for your breakfast, slice some carrots to grab on the go, have nuts or trail mix handy, make enough oatmeal or chia pudding for three or four days—and the list goes on and on.

HERBS AND FLOWER ESSENCES

One of the best ways to jumpstart healthy digestion, regulate appetite, and maintain regular bowel movements is to incorporate more bitter-tasting food, drinks, and herbs into your diet. Bitter herbs support digestion and liver health and should be a fundamental part of our diet. Include these in your daily or weekly routine to support digestion:

- → Blue vervain
- → Burdock root
- → Chamomile
- → Chicory
- → Damiana
- → Dandelion root and greens
- → Dark leafy greens like kale, mustard, or collards
- → Feverfew
- → Garden sage
- → Gentian
- → Lavender
- → Motherwort

The bitter taste starts a chain reaction that gets your entire digestive tract ready to work on breaking down and absorbing the food you eat. From the secretion of saliva when your mouth waters all the way through to your bowel movements, bitter herbs make every step of the digestion process work better. If you have trouble with poor appetite, sugar cravings, constipation, indigestion, sluggish digestion, or poor nutrient absorption, try incorporating bitter herbs and flavors into your daily and weekly routine.

Nowadays, we tend to cover up bitter flavors with sweet and/or creamy ones: the half-and-half we add to our coffee, the dairy and sugar we add to cacao to make milk chocolate, the creamy dressings we pour over our salads. These additions all distance our taste buds from the healing virtue of bitter. Instead, train your taste buds to appreciate the taste of bitter. Enjoy more salads with bitter greens, try your coffee black, buy a bar of dark chocolate, use apple cider or balsamic vinegars on your salad instead of creamy dressings, and make your own bitters formula to take before meals. The medicine of bitter herbs is in the taste, so stick to teas, tinctures, vinegars, and incorporating bitter foods into meals. A capsule will not do.

In addition to healthy digestion, bitter herbs help stimulate, cleanse, and protect the liver (helping with detoxification and elimination of toxins, which plays into skin health, hormone balancing, and more) while regulating blood sugar levels and curbing cravings.

Dandelion (*Taraxacum officinalis* and *T. erythrospermum*)

PARTS USED leaf, root

ENERGETICS cooling, drying

Both a nutritious food and powerful medicinal, dandelion is an admired herbal ally with a well-established history of use. A symbol of resiliency and perseverance, dandelion can often be seen bursting through concrete sidewalks and is found thriving in both sprawling cities and forests. A welcome sight for winter-weary humans and hungry pollinators, dandelion flowers are some of the first to bloom in early spring. Dandelion is high in vitamins A, B, and D, as well as minerals such as iron, potassium, calcium, and zinc.

Notable as a remedy for the digestive and urinary systems, dandelion has a restorative effect on both. Dandelion helps get the digestive juices flowing and promotes healthy elimination of waste. The leaf of dandelion is a well-loved spring tonic that can be added to salads or pesto, or sautéed with garlic and a squeeze of fresh lemon. A safe and effective diuretic, dandelion leaf tones the kidneys and aids in water elimination while maintaining proper potassium levels. The root is a digestive bitter and ally to the liver, stimulating bile flow that helps break down fats, alleviate indigestion, and detoxify while supporting healthy appetite and regular bowel movements. Like elecampane, the root of dandelion contains inulin, a known prebiotic that can help restore and support healthy gut flora.

WORD TO THE WISE The skin is the largest organ of elimination. When the liver, lymph, GI tract, and kidneys become overloaded by a buildup of toxins, excess hormones, inflammation, poor eating habits, and so on, the body will start to push toxins out through the skin. By supporting and cleansing the liver and entire digestive system with herbs like dandelion, we will often find relief from skin issues like eczema, dry skin, or acne, as well as relief from other conditions worsened by an overloaded liver, like PMS.

SUGGESTED PREPARATIONS Both the root and the leaf can be used in tea; the root is typically decocted for 10–15 minutes, the leaf can be simply steeped.

   ROOT: infusion or decoction, tincture, vinegar
   LEAF: salads, vinegar, tincture

FAVORITE PLANT PAIRINGS calendula, nettle, burdock, fennel, lemon balm

Roasted Dandelion Coffee Replacement

We might like coffee, but that doesn't always mean that coffee likes us. If stomach trouble, burnout, and jitters have you needing to give up your favorite morning ritual, turn to this herbal alternative. Roasted dandelion offers a similar taste without the afternoon crash. Together with roots like chicory and burdock, this blend supports the liver's detoxification process and promotes glowing skin, while ashwagandha replenishes the nervous, digestive, and endocrine systems that coffee depletes.

MAKES 4 CUPS OF TEA

> 3 tablespoons roasted dandelion
> 2 teaspoons ashwagandha
> 1 teaspoon chicory
> 1 teaspoon burdock
> 1 teaspoon cacao nibs

OPTIONAL: A few drops of gentian flower essence, a pinch of cinnamon and/or cardamom, coconut creamer or oat milk, a favorite herbal honey such as Hawthorn Rose Honey (page 149).
NOTE: All herbs should be cut and sifted. Leave out cacao nibs if trying to remove caffeine entirely.

To create this blend, add all the ingredients to a pint jar, put the lid on, and shake to combine. Label the jar with the tea name, ingredients, and date you made it. Store out of direct sunlight.

To prepare the brew, add 1 tablespoon of the blend per 8 ounces of water to a French press, a jar of your choice, or a reusable tea strainer. Cover and steep for 10–15 minutes, depending on desired strength. For an even more robust flavor, add filtered water to a small pot and bring to a gentle simmer. Add 1 tablespoon of the blend per 8 ounces of water to the pot and simmer, covered, for 5–10 minutes. Turn off the heat and steep, still covered, for an additional 5–10 minutes. Strain and serve with your favorite fixings.

Healthy Gut Flora, Healthy Immunity

At first glance, bacteria may seem more foe than friend. But we're finally realizing that there is good bacteria and harmful bacteria. There are bacteria that makes us sick and bacteria that help us stay well. It's when there's an imbalance in the amount of harmful bacteria that our health can be negatively affected. In fact, research suggests that as certain bad strains of bacteria take over, they can manipulate your cravings so you continue to want the very food that sustains their growth, thus keeping you unwell.

> There are bacteria that makes us sick and bacteria that help us stay well. It's when there's an imbalance in the amount of harmful bacteria that our health can be negatively affected.

To keep your immune system functioning optimally, consider your gut health, and in particular, your gut flora. This flora, part of your microbiome, comprises a whole host of microorganisms that ensure your vitality. Some of these microorganisms act in a mutualistic way, aiding your body in essential functioning such as synthesizing vitamins B and K and supporting the immune system in protecting against infection. Healthy gut flora discourages pathogens, decreases inflammation, and modulates immune health.

LIFESTYLE

The key to maintaining happy gut flora and a well-functioning immune system is a good diet. Make healthy eating a priority. First make sure you're getting plenty of fiber in the form of colorful vegetables, whole grains, and medicinal roots. Consider an anti-inflammatory diet (page 66) and removing any foods that may be stressing your immune system and digestion. Get a daily dose of fermented foods. Too much sugar, caffeine, alcohol, or other common food triggers like dairy, gluten, soy, nightshades, and corn can cause inflammation, gas, bloating, heartburn, and the like, so avoid these foods or eliminate them altogether.

Making Your Own Sauerkraut

Fermented foods like sauerkraut, kimchi, kombucha, yogurt and lacto-fermented veggies, and homemade ginger beer pack a probiotic punch, thereby creating healthy gut flora and proper digestion. Making it at home is easy, empowering, and a whole lot more affordable than buying it at the grocery store. It also gives you an opportunity to engage in fun kitchen projects (page 48) that result in delicious foods and fizzy beverages that benefit your gut, foster immunity, and delight your taste buds. This sauerkraut recipe is inspired by fermenter Sandor Katz.

MAKES 4 CUPS

> 2 pounds cabbage
> 1 tablespoon salt, adding more if need be
> If available, add fresh, chopped nettle leaf, violet leaf, calendula petals, and/or lemon balm, or more conventional seasoning like dried (or fresh) dill or caraway seeds.
> Wide-mouth quart jar or fermentation crock
> Medium- to large-size mixing bowl

To start, remove the outer leaves of the cabbage, washing without peeling any other layers. Depending on the consistency you want for your finished product, roughly chop or grate all the cabbage into a bowl.

Once chopped and in the bowl, sprinkle and mix salt and other seasonings or chopped fresh herbs into the cabbage. Sauerkraut doesn't require a lot of salt, but go ahead and taste and see if more is needed. Using your hands to mix and gently massage ingredients together for this step is fine.

Once salted and seasoned to your preference, begin to firmly massage and squeeze the cabbage for a few minutes. The point is to break down the cell walls and release the water from the cabbage, fresh herbs, or other veggies. This liquid, or brine, will be what the cabbage mixture is submerged in during the fermentation process, so there should be a decent amount. Fermentation expert Sandor Katz suggests you should be able to pick up a handful of cabbage and have it drip with liquid, much like a wet sponge.

From there, pack the cabbage mixture and brine into a quart jar. Press down with force on the mixture, packing it in with fingers or a blunt tool. You want to get rid of any air pockets while the brine rises and fully covers the cabbage mix. Fill the jar just about to the top, leaving some space (half an inch or so) for expansion. Keep the cabbage mix fully submerged in the brine the entire time, so use a smaller jar, a small glass or ceramic insert (made specifically for this), or a clean rock to press the mix down, or you can use the outer cabbage leaves folded to fit in the jar.

Screw on the lid and keep the kraut in a warm, dry spot in the kitchen—above the fridge, next to a window, or in a cabinet. Depending on the taste desired and the climate where you live, this process can take 3 days to a few months. Warmer weather means less fermentation time. If you like a stronger-tasting kraut, you'll want to let it sit longer.

Begin sampling your kraut a few days in. When it gets to your preferred taste and consistency (the cabbage will lose its crunchiness the longer it ferments) it's ready.

HERBS AND FLOWER ESSENCES

Many of you are already familiar with probiotics—foods such as yogurt, sauerkraut, miso, or kimchi; or probiotic supplements that are alive with strains of good-for-you bacteria and yeast that improves digestive functioning, immune health, and overall well-being.

As it turns out, these microorganisms require their own source of sustenance to maintain their equilibrium once you've ingested them. This sustenance is known as a *prebiotic*, a form of dietary fiber that your gut flora feeds off of. A diet of processed foods, sugary snacks and drinks, not enough fiber, and few fruits and vegetables will make for poor digestion, very little beneficial gut flora, and a weak immune system. Fortunately, many medicinal herbs and grocery store staples are packed with fiber. In particular, inulin, one type of dietary fiber, has been shown to help rebuild healthy gut flora. Higher amounts of inulin and other types of dietary fiber can be found in the following herbs, foods, and grains:

→ Apples

→ Asparagus

→ Barley

→ Burdock root

→ Chicory root

→ Dandelion root and leaf

→ Elecampane root

→ Flaxseed

→ Garlic

→ Jerusalem artichoke

→ Leeks

→ Oats

→ Onions

→ Seaweeds

→ Wheat

Drink any of these herbs in daily infusions, add them to your meals, and eat lots of the fibrous fruits and veggies listed above to support your immunity, gut flora, digestive health, and overall well-being.

Ginger (*Zingiber officinale*)

PARTS USED root

ENERGETICS warming, drying

Ginger is a wonderfully warming herb that plays an indispensable role in stoking the digestive fire, relieving pain and inflammation throughout the body, and supporting us when we're sick with a cold or flu. In fact, ginger reminds us that the food we eat is medicine and that the medicine we take in can be delicious and enjoyable.

As you sip ginger tea you'll notice that the warmth in your core begins to radiate outward, bringing circulation and warmth to your limbs as well. In this way ginger helps you relax and release tension. Think about what your body does when you get into a nice warm bath. As you exhale deeply, your muscles loosen and you are present and calm. But what about stepping outside on a freezing cold day or taking a swim in a cold river? Your body tends to tense up as you pull yourself inward and contract. Like a nice warm bath, ginger uncoils the tension we carry and opens us up so we feel more vibrant.

Ginger can relieve pain by increasing circulation and reducing inflammation, and it can shift patterns of tension and cold when added to a bath or foot soak, infused and added to a massage or body oil, or taken as tea. If you have delayed menstruation, clots, or menstrual cramps, try working with a hot ginger infusion or warm ginger compress on your abdomen. If you are stiff and sore from overwork or a chronic condition like arthritis, try using ginger body oil or salve topically as well as adding ginger to your meals or favorite herbal tea by bringing warmth to one's core, ginger is one of the best herbs for promoting healthy digestion. Symptoms of poor digestion include gas, bloating, constipation, feeling heavy after meals, or a white coating on the tongue. Try incorporating ginger into your meals or sip ginger tea afterward to promote digestion and calm. Ginger is an excellent remedy for those with cold hands and feet, poor circulation, and a tendency to feel chilled, especially when feeling under the weather. Additionally, it is an antimicrobial and can offer relief from a sore throat and prevent further infection.

WORD TO THE WISE A tried-and-true remedy for motion sickness, ginger settles the stomach and stabilizes the senses. The efficacy of ginger for preventing nausea, dizziness, and vomiting—whether due to travel, conventional cancer treatment, or pregnancy—is renowned and well researched.

SUGGESTED PREPARATIONS herbal honey, hot infusion, broth, stir-fry, body oil

FAVORITE PLANT PAIRINGS elderberry, holy basil/tulsi, elecampane, gotu kola, lemon balm

Ginger Lemon Infusion

This simple and effective infusion can be enjoyed all winter long to help fight off infection, support liver and digestive health, and bring circulation to the arms, legs, hands, and feet.

MAKES 4 CUPS

1 inch knob of fresh ginger, sliced or grated
1 whole lemon, cut into thin slices

Put the ingredients in a quart jar or French press. Bring 32 ounces of water to a boil and pour it over the blend and allow it to steep for a minimum of 15 minutes. You may wish to add a tablespoon of herbal or local raw honey and/or a splash of your favorite bourbon or rye for an extra kick. Drink it hot and sip throughout the day.

Stress and Digestion

Have you ever had an intense conversation over a meal that left you feeling bloated or gassy, or with an uncomfortable feeling in the stomach? Or how about that first date when you were overcome with nerves and barely ate, even though you were starving before you met up? These are just a few examples of the interplay between your digestive system and your nervous system. One way the gut and brain are connected is through the stress response. When we experience a stressor, the fight-flight-freeze response kicks in, shifting the body's priorities. Think about it: from an evolutionary perspective, when people experienced a stressor or threat—say, being charged by a wild animal—it was time to bolt, not time to sit down and enjoy a meal.

Without a healthy gut and well-functioning digestive system, the vitamins and minerals in our food are not properly absorbed, and we may experience skin issues like acne or eczema, a sluggish immune response to pathogens, and improper function of important neurotransmitters and hormones. Moreover, since the gut and the brain are connected, poor gut function affects mood and memory. If you eat poorly, experience chronic stress, or repeatedly eat a food known to cause inflammation or irritation, chances are not only will your physical health suffer, but so will your mental and emotional well-being.

LIFESTYLE

Digestion requires a lot of energy. When your awareness is focused on issues that cause minor or major stress, whether it be an argument with a loved one at the dinner table, a boss who doesn't respect your lunch break, or scrolling through social media or reacting to the news while eating, you'll likely find that your appetite is diminished or that your food is not properly digested, meaning you won't absorb the nutrients in your food and you'll experience gas, bloating, or heartburn. That's why it's crucial to set aside time to enjoy meals. In an ideal world, we'd all have time to prepare three meals a day and grow small, abundant gardens in our yards or on our windowsills. But barring that, there are things you can do to lessen stress, create sacred space around mealtime, and thereby support healthy digestion.

For instance, did you know that digestion begins before your first bite of food, with the link between your sense of smell and your salivary glands? Think about the last time you walked into a restaurant or arrived home to find a loved one preparing a meal. The smell of sautéed onions and garlic alone can instigate a chain reaction that gets your mouth watering and your digestive juices flowing, all while your stomach begins to growl in hungry anticipation, preparing your body to break down and assimilate the meal ahead.

Even if you aren't preparing the meal, if you're eating leftovers or grabbing a quick snack, you can aid your digestion and shift out of stress mode by pausing for a moment and taking a deep breath in and smelling the food in front of you. You'll notice you immediately begin to salivate, and you'll feel more settled in your body as you switch from the busyness of your day to the calmer, more centered, rest-and-digest state that is necessary for proper digestion.

Beyond that, take care to remove any foods that could be causing your digestive and nervous systems undue stress. These are the foods that are highly processed or cause inflammation. Try removing or lessening your intake of alcohol, sugar, dairy, red meat, and gluten while increasing your intake of colorful fresh fruits and vegetables.

PRACTICE: EATING MINDFULLY

Redefining your relationship with food can be extremely empowering, and it starts with being mindful. Let's talk about what it means to eat mindfully. Mindful eating is just as much about how you're eating your food, where it came from, and how it was prepared as it is about what you're eating. Are you eating with a sense of shame and guilt, each bite bringing up feelings of inadequacy? Are you eating on autopilot, grabbing whatever is in front of you without pausing or savoring? Do you consider your impact on the environment when you shop for groceries? When we're talking about mindfulness, whether in terms of the food we eat or our new meditation practice, it's all about bringing a sense of awareness into what we do.

As you develop a relationship with your body and the food you eat, remember to move forward with curiosity and compassion. Many of us have deeply personal relationships with food, and it may take time to shift eating habits. There will be good days and bad, but the bad days don't mean we're bad people. It's not about overnight results; it's about daily practices that prioritize whatever a healthy diet looks like for you. This isn't about shaming yourself because you ate ice cream; it's about taking ownership of your needs and making informed, empowering choices. An empowered choice could be a bowl of ice cream or large popcorn at the movies, as these foods can bring us joy, feel like a treat, and satiate a craving; or it could be a big glass of water and a perfectly cooked veggie bowl. Mindful eating is about fully engaging with the food you love, being conscious of any stories or patterns you carry around food, and developing a healthy awareness of what nourishes you and brings you joy in the long term.

PRACTICE: FOOD JOURNALING

Pay attention to which foods nourish you and which foods make you feel the worse for wear. A great way to keep track of how your food makes you feel, especially if you're trying to better understand your body, moods, and underlying health issues, is to keep a food journal. This isn't about counting calories or obsessing over food intake; it's about noticing, without judging yourself, and how your food choices impact your overall health.

Maybe your energy levels are more consistent throughout the day when you start your morning with a big glass of water and some herbal tea instead of coffee. Or you realize the day after you eat a lot of dairy you always get a migraine, but you've never put two and two together. Maybe when you eat out at certain restaurants your digestion tends to feel off. You'll be amazed at how things like headaches, PMS, anxiety, blood sugar levels, acne, and more chronic issues like autoimmune disorders, depression, arthritis, irritable bowel syndrome, and allergies can be affected for better or worse by the foods you eat. You'll never really know until you pay attention! That's where food journaling comes in.

Helpful Guidelines for Food Journaling

→ Keep your journal with you or make notes in your phone.

→ You don't have to show anyone, so be honest and real.

→ Make a note of what you eat and drink immediately after you're done eating so you don't forget.

→ Make note of your stress level, mood, or any thoughts or feelings going on before, during, and after you eat or drink.

→ Write a positive affirmation about your body, your journey with food, your health, etc. Make it personal and relevant. This is about gratitude for your process, awareness, and insight, and not about shame and self-judgment.

HERBS AND FLOWER ESSENCES

Herbal medicine is incredibly well-suited to addressing stress, poor digestion, and the effects of an unhealthy diet. Stress and digestive ailments are among the most common health complaints today. Many of the herbs discussed in this book that help with sleep, relaxation, pain relief, vitality, and focus also have an affinity for soothing, strengthening, and supporting both the digestive and the nervous systems for optimal health and resiliency.

Since the sense of smell plays an important role in encouraging healthy digestion, just as it does in cultivating a state of relaxation and calm, there are no better herbs to work with when targeting both your mood and your digestive health than those with potent aromatics. These include:

- → Chamomile
- → Cinnamon
- → Coriander
- → Fennel
- → Garden basil
- → Garden sage
- → Ginger
- → Holy basil/tulsi
- → Lavender
- → Lemon balm
- → Meadowsweet
- → Mints (peppermint, spearmint, catnip)
- → Rosemary
- → Thyme

Aromatic herbs—what herbalists call *carminative* herbs—are fragrant, volatile, oil-rich plants that offer a host of healing benefits. We often think of these as culinary herbs, but don't let that fool you—these herbs won't just delight your taste buds, they each carry their own unique healing powers. Aromatic herbs assist with indigestion, battle mental fatigue and brain fog, soothe inflammation, calm tired nerves, uplift mood, relax an anxious mind, and are strongly antimicrobial. Try sipping fennel ginger tea after a heavy meal, or blend a stress-reducing digestive tea using chamomile, catnip, ginger, and holy basil/tulsi. You can also incorporate a whole range of aromatic herbs into the meals you love.

If you want to work with a flower essence for combating stress and supporting digestion, try wild rose or devil's claw to start. Wild rose is an excellent essence when you feel resigned to a life of stress and digestive problems and need a helping hand to motivate and encourage positive changes. Devil's claw can be helpful for those of us who lack self-awareness and self-esteem. So often we take in messages about our diet, body image, health, and confidence level from the world around us. Our bodies become a battleground, and we never learn who we really are without the gaze or opinions of others. Devil's claw allows you to engage with your true nature, to anchor into yourself, practice mindfulness and intuitive eating, and decipher which habits and qualities empower you.

Catnip (*Nepeta cataria*)

PARTS USED leaves

ENERGETICS cool, dry

A mint family plant, catnip is versatile and dependable. Catnip reminds us that there is no separation between body and mind, offering calm and relief whenever stress and digestive woes impact us.

A curative staple for centuries, catnip has been used in European folk medicine to reduce stress and upset in both the nervous and digestive systems. Like most aromatic and bitter medicinal plants, catnip is a prime example of an herb's ability to work on these two systems simultaneously. Catnip brings the body into a rest-and-digest state naturally and gently, and out of an overly stressed, fight-flight-freeze state. If digestive distress tends to start up or intensify when you're under stress, incorporate catnip into your routine. Likewise, if you tend to be so stressed that you lose your appetite or live in your head, forgetting to eat, a cup of catnip, damiana, and chamomile tea can bring you back to life, easing nervousness and tension while awakening your digestive system and renewing your hunger. Catnip allows you to set aside the weight of whatever has you feeling anxious or irritated so that you can be present, enjoy a meal, and relax a little. Catnip can also offer support if you have issues with body image or disordered eating, encouraging intuitive eating and mindfulness around mealtime.

WORD TO THE WISE If rats or mosquitoes are plaguing your garden, patio area, or compost bin, try growing catnip around the perimeter to help ward either off, as they dislike the plant and will not approach. Traditionally catnip was grown alongside fields and around areas of grain storage for protection against rats. In addition, catnip can also repel mosquitoes more effectively than many insect repellents and is a fragrant, easy-to-grow alternative.

SUGGESTED PREPARATIONS hot infusion, tincture

FAVORITE PLANT PAIRINGS fennel, chamomile, skullcap, lemon balm

Trust Your Gut Infusion

Turn to this herbal infusion when you are rattled or feeling overwhelmed by a decision, if you are stressed and anxious with thoughts looping around in your head and knots in your stomach, perhaps experiencing digestive unease like gas, bloating, heaviness, or stomach cramps. This tea will soothe your upset stomach and bring clarity and stillness to the decision-making process.

MAKES 4 CUPS

1 tablespoon wood betony
1 tablespoon gotu kola
1 tablespoon lemon balm
3 teaspoons catnip
2 teaspoons dandelion root
2 teaspoons licorice root
1 teaspoon fennel

NOTE: All herbs should be cut and sifted.

To make the tea blend, add all ingredients to a small jar, put a lid on, and shake thoroughly to combine. Label the jar with the blend title, ingredients, and date you made it. Store the blend out of direct sunlight and it will keep for 8 months to a year.

When ready to prepare this tea, use 1 heaping tablespoon of the blend for every 8 ounces of water. For 1 serving, add 1 tablespoon to a reusable tea strainer or place in a jar or cup, cover with boiling water, and steep for a minimum of 15 minutes, the longer the more potent the infusion. For brewing up to 32 ounces, add the blend to a glass jar or French press, cover with boiling water, and allow to steep for 5–15 minutes. Drink hot or refrigerate and enjoy chilled.

Gut Inflammation and Digestive Distress

With all that the GI tract does, you can bet you'll need to step in from time to time and do some maintenance. These days it's rare to encounter someone who doesn't have some sort of digestive complaint. Sadly, the standard American diet—abbreviated, ironically, as SAD—is marked by overly processed, artificially sweetened, and refined foods; sugary drinks; caffeine; and too much fried food, alcohol, and red meat. It has been shown to wreak havoc on digestion, abusing the gut lining and straining one's overall health. When poor eating is coupled with a high-stress lifestyle, the result is serious: ulcers, heartburn, acid reflux, poor nutrient absorption, skin issues, and depleted beneficial gut flora. Poor gut health has been linked to chronic issues like autoimmune disorders, brain fog, fatigue, depression, anxiety, food allergies and sensitivities, type 2 diabetes, irritable bowel syndrome, and heart disease, to name a few.

LIFESTYLE

Cleaning up your diet and managing your stress levels is a great place to start to restore digestive health, though you may want to work with herbs that combat the inflammation caused by poor eating habits, thereby promoting deeper healing. This is especially important if you've been dealing with longstanding digestive issues or major health concerns.

Think of your gut lining much like you would your skin. If you get a cut or scrape on your skin, you can try not to touch it and be proactive about using first-aid herbs and a bandage to quicken healing time—or you can continue to rough around, working against your body's attempts to heal itself, meaning the cut or scrape will heal more slowly and perhaps become infected or lead to scarring. Gut healing works the same way. If you continue to eat a poor diet with processed foods and not drink enough water, your gut health will suffer, resulting in long-term issues that will take longer to heal. Shifting to a good diet along with incorporating gut-healing herbs like aloe, calendula, chamomile, licorice, marshmallow, meadowsweet, plantain, and violet leaf will aid in your healing process and restore gut health.

PRACTICE: REDUCE INFLAMMATION

Going on an anti-inflammatory diet for six to eight weeks while limiting or eliminating the amount of inflammatory foods you eat (e.g., gluten, sugar, caffeine, alcohol, dairy, and soy, as well as nightshades like tomatoes, potatoes, eggplant, peppers, red spices, etc.) can be a great first step in healing your gut.

Anti-inflammatory diets usually focus on upping the amount of whole, fresh vegetables and fruits you eat while emphasizing lean meats, healthy fats, nuts, and seeds. After six to eight weeks on this diet, you can try reintroducing one food group per week and see how your body responds. For example, if you've really been missing your morning coffee, brew a cup and notice what happens. You'll want to pay attention to not only how you're feeling immediately after drinking your coffee but also for the rest of the day and the next few days. Maybe you won't notice much, so you might carry on with your morning coffee practice. However, perhaps after reintroducing coffee you find your anxiety spikes, your regular bowel movements go off, you get a dull headache, or you realize that when you drink coffee you forget to eat or drink water. These insights can empower you to make the best choices for your health instead of being on autopilot.

Along with dietary adjustments, taking medicinal herbs that support gut health can make a huge difference in healing even longstanding, chronic issues. Once your body has time to clear and reset, you may notice that symptoms like brain fog, gas, bloating, moodiness, anxiety, fatigue, general sluggishness, ulcers, irritable bowel syndrome, and/or apathy begin to dissipate or lessen.

> *Anti-inflammatory diets usually focus on upping the amount of whole, fresh vegetables and fruits you eat while emphasizing lean meats, healthy fats, nuts, and seeds.*

This is an excellent time to start a food journal and practice mindful eating (page 60) to bring awareness to how you feel as a result of what you eat. At the very least, removing inflammatory foods will offer you a better understanding of your body so that you can make conscious choices about the foods you eat.

Herb-infused, inflammation-reducing meals don't have to be complicated. At first it might seem a little daunting to remove so many food staples from your diet. Many of us can't imagine not eating gluten (wheat, rye, barley) or dairy, but if digestive distress, immune system problems, and mood-related complaints are a constant for you, trying an anti-inflammatory diet for six to eight weeks can be truly life changing. Use this chart for insight and inspiration (and remember, components of each meal, like roasted veggies, can be prepared ahead of time on your prep day). In addition, check out the resources (page 241) for cookbook recommendations.

Anti-Inflammatory Meals

BREAKFAST	LUNCH	DINNER	SNACKS
overnight oats with nuts, seeds, and berries	spicy chicken lettuce wraps	fish of choice with asparagus and lemon	chia seed pudding with strawberries, coconut milk, cinnamon, marshmallow root, ashwagandha, and cocoa powder
scrambled eggs, sautéed fresh greens (chard, spinach, kale, etc.), and shiitake mushrooms with herb-infused vinegar	crispy tofu spring rolls with fresh basil and mint	rice bowl with kidney or black beans, steamed broccoli, greens, and roasted squash	popcorn with nettle and nori gomasio on top
ginger congee with fried eggs and green onions	salad with romaine and other leafy greens, protein of choice (nuts, seeds, meat, chickpeas), and oil and vinegar dressing	curried butternut squash soup with pumpkin seeds on top	trail mix with almonds, walnuts, pecans, cashews, and dried fruit like cherries, goji berries, raisins
roasted sweet potato hash, bacon, gluten-free toast with nettle and chickweed pesto	salad with roasted cauliflower and carrots, protein of choice (nuts, seeds, meat, chickpeas), and tahini dressing	shrimp or pork shoulder tacos with corn tortillas and lots of toppings like sliced radish, pickled onions, cilantro, lime, and salsa	veggies and/or corn chips with hummus

HERBS AND FLOWER ESSENCES

The use of herbs for gut healing can vary from person to person, depending on the complaint and how severe. Generally, you will want to use herbs to both soothe inflammation and repair the gut lining. Daily use of chamomile is ideal for GI complaints, as it reduces inflammation, fights infection, calms spasms and cramps, and dispels gas and bloating while being gentle enough for all ages. In addition, licorice, marshmallow root, plantain, calendula, and meadowsweet are extremely handy herbal allies for gut healing.

The best way to work with herbs for gut healing will be drinking herbal infusions on a daily basis. Infusions, more potent than herbal teas due to a longer brewing time, bring the healing plant constituents into direct contact with inflamed, damaged tissue in the GI tract. Try making a quart of Trust Your Gut Infusion (page 64) daily for half the week, and prepare Marshmallow Cold Infusion (page 70) every day for the other half. Remember, consistency is key.

If you want to work with flower essences, try black-eyed Susan and impatiens. Black-eyed Susan encourages us to notice habits and beliefs that hold us back and keep us in unhealthy patterns, away from true self-awareness. This essence aids us in acknowledging the hard work we must do to heal ourselves and can be helpful if you are having trouble giving up certain habits that negatively affect your digestion or overall health. Impatiens flower essence can be used when healing long-term, chronic issues that require patience and dedication. Gut-healing won't happen overnight, and this essence will help to quell impatience or frustration during the long process.

Marshmallow (*Althaea officinalis*)

PARTS USED mostly root, though leaves and flowers can be used

ENERGETICS cooling, moistening

A favorite of mine, and an essential plant for many herbalists, marshmallow is an outstanding remedy for soothing the mucous membranes of the gastrointestinal, urinary, and respiratory tracts and can be used topically to treat inflamed, dry skin. A relative of hibiscus and hollyhock, marshmallow is a demulcent (soothing) herb with delicate, soft flowers. The root is most often used and commercially available, though if the leaves and flowers are available, they can be used with the same results. Demulcent herbs produce a cooling, inflammation-reducing mucilage that coats the tissues, bringing relief to a painful sore throat or longstanding digestive distress. A mildly sweet, nutritive infusion, marshmallow offers immediate hydration when feeling dry and brittle. When demulcent, mucilage-rich herbs like mallow are ingested, they create a moistening effect throughout the body and can be safely enjoyed daily to hydrate us from the inside out.

A remedy for leaky gut, ulcers, constipation, and irritable bowel syndrome, marshmallow works wonders on the stomach and intestines when incorporated into a daily self-care practice. When there is irritation and inflammation in the gastrointestinal tract, nutrients may not be absorbed efficiently, leading to fatigue or further physical or mood-related imbalances. Consider mallow a foundational herb for constitutionally dry types who are prone to chronic illness and inflammation.

A quart of Marshmallow Cold Infusion (page 70) daily is recommended for painful, inflamed urinary tract infections. Whereas elecampane is for cold, heavy respiratory conditions with phlegm (page 179), marshmallow is recommended when you have a dry cough and a scratchy throat. Marshmallow works in the same manner as slippery elm and makes an ideal substitute, as slippery elm is currently on United Plant Savers At-Risk list.

WORD TO THE WISE If you tend toward dry, red skin, take an oatmeal and marshmallow root bath by adding a few handfuls of oatstraw or oatmeal and a tablespoon or two of marshmallow root to the water. You could even add some calendula flowers and rose petals. If this issue is more localized to your face, perhaps due to a harsh, dry winter, try using the Honey Mallow Soothing Face Mask (page 71).

SUGGESTED PREPARATIONS cold infusion or powdered and added to oatmeal, ghee, or honey

FAVORITE PLANT PAIRINGS chamomile, rose, plantain, calendula

Marshmallow Cold Infusion

This simple brew is perfect to soothe and cool inflamed, dry tissue. Consider it a daily staple if you are trying to restore GI tract health; if you have an ulcer, heartburn, or other digestive distress; or if you feel chronically dry, with dry mouth, lips, hair, skin, or nails.

MAKES 4 CUPS

4 tablespoons marshmallow root (cut)

Add the marshmallow root to a quart jar and fill with cool or room-temperature water. Let steep for a minimum of 15 minutes, though an overnight infusion is best. Strain and sip throughout the day.

OPTIONAL: Place marshmallow root in a small, reusable cloth tea bag and put in the quart jar with water. Steeping time is the same. Before you're ready to drink, massage the bag to get out as much mucilage-rich goo as possible.

Honey Mallow Soothing Face Mask

This beneficial treatment alleviates inflamed, dry, itchy skin. Apply this as an all-over facial mask or as a spot treatment on acne, eczema, or irritated skin anywhere on the body.

MAKES ½ CUP

> ½ cup local raw honey
> 3 tablespoons powdered marshmallow root
> 1 tablespoon powdered oats
> 1 teaspoon powdered rose petals
> 1 teaspoon powdered chamomile and/or calendula
> **OPTIONAL:** 1 teaspoon green clay or powdered plantain leaf

To create the mask, simply mix together the honey and powdered herbs in a small jar. The herbs can be purchased already powdered or whole herbs can be blended in a spice grinder. If need be, gently warm the honey before adding to the jar. To do this, fill a small pot with an inch or two of water and place the honey jar in it. Slowly heat on the stovetop, stirring the honey with a chopstick or knife until it's liquid and easier to pour. *Do not overheat raw honey or bring water to a boil*. Once the honey is pourable, combine with the powdered herbs in the jar. Stir into a paste and allow the honey to cool to room temperature. Feel free to add a pinch more of any ingredient if you're wanting a thicker consistency. Label the face mask with the ingredients and the date you made it.

To use the mask, apply it liberally to your face or trouble area. Leave for 10–15 minutes and up to 30 minutes. This recipe will make enough for 5 or 6 facial mask treatments, as a little goes a long way. Store in a cool place in your bathroom or in the fridge and it will keep for 12–18 months.

Calendula (*Calendula officinalis*)

PARTS USED flower

ENERGETICS cooling, drying

Guided by the warming rays of the sun, calendula is a versatile, brightly hued, golden-orange flower that grows abundantly throughout the summer months. Renowned for its topical benefits, calendula should not be overlooked for internal complaints as well. Notably, calendula has an affinity for healing the lining of the gut, soothing the GI tract, and easing longstanding inflammation and digestive distress that results from a poor diet. Complaints like ulcers, gas, bloating, and autoimmune issues can all benefit from this vibrant herb.

When problematic foods are removed from the diet, calendula is able to aid in bringing the body's overactive inflammatory response into balance, clearing stagnation by supporting the healthy movement of lymph and cleansing the blood, keeping channels of elimination open and detoxifying waste products.

Lethargy, mild depression, and melancholy have increasingly been related to inflammation caused by troublesome dietary choices. Calendula gently brightens your mood while getting to the root of the problem and bringing greater healing.

When taken internally as a tea or tincture—or my personal favorite, combined with violet and cleavers and massaged on the skin as an infused oil—calendula supports healthy lymph movement, which can be especially supportive for chronic health concerns when there is general fatigue and a feeling of heaviness and cold, as well as tenderness and swelling in the lymph nodes.

Lastly, for topical use, calendula is beloved as a first-aid ally for all manner of bumps and bruises. This plant's ability to heal wounds, stop bleeding, reduce the redness and soreness of bruises, and fight bacterial and fungal infection proves what an exceptional curative calendula is. In addition, calendula is a principal herb for general skin care, as it is rich in antioxidants and generous in its ability to tone and tighten as well as soothe dry, inflamed skin for all manner of facial and body-care needs.

WORD TO THE WISE Calendula thrives as a potted herb and can make a wonderful addition to any home garden. For medicinal potency, pick the flowers just as they begin to bloom and open—a gardening technique called *deadheading*.

SUGGESTED PREPARATIONS infused oil, hot infusion, tincture

FAVORITE PLANT PAIRINGS marshmallow, chamomile, violet, rose, ginger

Gut-Healing Infusion

An herbal infusion for a happy gut, this preparation is packed with some of the best gut-healing herbs that help soothe inflammation, repair damaged GI tract tissue, and provide support for chronic issues that have a digestive component such as autoimmune disorders. You'll gain the best results if 3–4 cups are enjoyed as a daily tonic for an extended period of time, 4–6 weeks or longer, depending on the complaint.

MAKES 4 CUPS OF TEA

2 tablespoons calendula
2 tablespoons meadowsweet
1 tablespoon gotu kola
2 teaspoons chamomile
1 teaspoon rose petals

NOTE: All herbs should be cut and sifted.

To create this infusion, combine the ingredients in a pint jar, put the lid on, and shake until mixed. Label the jar with the blend name, ingredients, and the date you made it. Store it out of direct sunlight and it will keep for 12–18 months.

When ready to drink, add 1 tablespoon of the blend per 8 ounces of water to a jar, French press, or favorite mug or reusable tea strainer. Bring the water to a boil, pour over the blend, and allow to steep for a minimum of 15 minutes, longer for a more potent infusion. Reheat if need be or sip chilled over ice and enjoy!

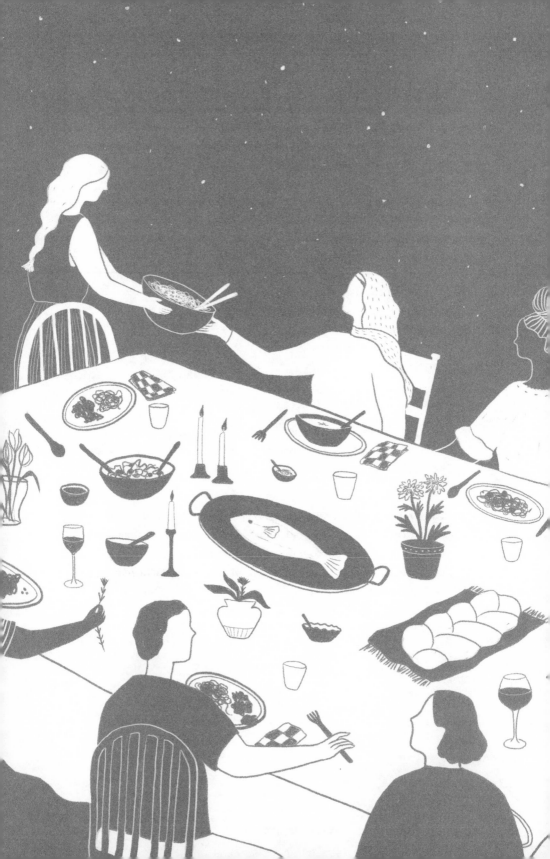

Vitality and Mental Clarity

4

AS DISCUSSED IN CHAPTER 3, diet and digestion are fundamental to your ability to experience well-being while being the cornerstone of your body's nutrition. Nutrient deficiencies, poor diet, lack of exercise, and a high-stress lifestyle, all increasingly common today, impact not only the digestive system but one's overall vitality, affecting energy levels, mental clarity, and the ability to focus and retain information. Improving your diet and digestive health is an essential place to start for any health concern, but if you are also experiencing issues with your energy levels, focus, and memory, there are many herbs and practices that can help.

In this chapter we will focus on two groups of herbs, nutritives and adaptogens, which both build on the healing work of chapter 3 while also supporting memory, mental clarity, focus, and overall vitality. These herbs, often categorized as restorative tonics, when taken on a daily basis, can improve your stress response, sleep, memory, mood, and energy levels, as well as support immune modulation and function; more efficient elimination and detoxification; and stronger nails, skin, and hair.

NUTRITIVES

Of all the herbs, some of my absolute favorites for personal use, as well as my most recommended, are the nutritive herbs. Most of us are nutrient deficient, which leads to complaints like fatigue, poor focus, depression, stress, low immunity, pain, and other chronic issues. Herbalists work with nutritives, which are affordable, easily absorbable, and nutrient-dense whole herbs, to remedy a host of problems and increase the amount of vitamins and minerals you take in.

Although most herbs carry some nutritional value, herbs considered nutritive are more concentrated, containing higher quantities of a specific vitamin or mineral. For example, rose hips are an excellent source of vitamin C, and nettle contains high levels of iron and calcium, as well as magnesium, potassium, chlorophyll, and silica. Even better, nutritive herbs are safe to use for almost everyone, can and even should be consumed in large quantities, and are easy to find commercially or growing near you.

Nutritives are especially useful when we have deficiencies that require a higher dose of vitamins and minerals. Common deficiencies include magnesium, calcium, vitamin D, iron, and the B vitamins like B_{12} and folic acid. Sure, you can take a multivitamin, but instead of relying on a costly supplement that your body doesn't recognize as food and may or may not absorb, it's more efficient and a lot more empowering to add fresh or dried nettle leaf to your pesto; make an iron-rich syrup with powerhouses like dandelion, nettle, and rose hips; or drink a deep, emerald-hued overnight infusion of nettle, oatstraw, and alfalfa. See the chart on page 78 for more ideas.

Since we could all use a little assistance getting a nutritional boost to our diet, why not create a relationship with these plants? Many nutritive herbs are also considered vital wild food sources, making working with them a great way to reestablish ancestral food and medicine traditions to honor your lineage.

Although most herbs carry some nutritional value, herbs considered nutritive are more concentrated, containing higher qualities of a specific vitamin or mineral.

Getting the Most Out of Nutritive Herbs

Working with your favorite nutritive herbs can be fun and easy, but it does require a little know-how. Certain preparations are better for getting the vitamins and minerals from the plant into your body. When trying to get the most out of these nutritive herbs, you'll want to eat the herbs, incorporating them—fresh, dried, or powdered—into broths, salt blends, pestos, salads, smoothies, soups, and stir-fries. You can also try water-based preparations such as cold or hot infusions (page 221) and decoctions (page 223). Remember, an infusion requires a much longer steeping time than your typical cup of tea, especially when it comes to nutritive herbs. Steep your nutritive herbal infusions for a few hours and up to overnight to extract the most nutrients out of the herb.

Tinctures, which are alcohol based, are great for ingesting certain helpful plant constituents but aren't ideal for extracting vitamins and minerals. Instead, stick with water preparations mentioned above or experiment with herbal vinegars and oxymels (page 231). Oxymels are medicine with a honey and vinegar base; and herbal vinegars are better than alcohol when wanting to work with high vitamin and mineral plants but, similar to tinctures, can be kept in a dropper bottle and carried with you for easy use.

Nutritives

NUTRIENT	HERBAL SOURCE
VITAMIN C	rose hips, alfalfa, violet leaf, hibiscus
CALCIUM	nettle, oatstraw, dandelion leaf, red clover
IRON	dandelion leaf and root, nettle, chickweed, burdock root, marshmallow root
MAGNESIUM	oatstraw, nettle, dandelion root, burdock root, cacao/dark chocolate, red clover
POTASSIUM	oatstraw, nettle, dandelion leaf and root, red clover, alfalfa

ADAPTOGENS

As you replenish and build up your intake of vitamins and minerals with nutritives, a class of herbs called *adaptogens* helps modulate any systems that aren't working their best while focusing on nourishing the adrenals. Often declared to be cure-alls and miracle plants, this group of herbs has been receiving a lot of attention lately for their ability to boost energy and promote endurance and vitality. Adaptogens aid your body by helping you adapt to all that life throws your way. Sounds pretty great, right? The term is relatively new, having been coined in the 1940s by scientists who were, among other things, interested in these plants for their ability to override mental and physical exhaustion. However, these herbs have been respected and revered for hundreds and even thousands of years.

The following adaptogenic herbs have a longstanding history of use in Traditional Chinese Medicine, Ayurveda, and Cherokee medicine as herbs that improve vital force, sustain energy, and maintain optimal health:

→ Ashwagandha (page 84)

→ Ginseng, American

→ Ginseng, Asian

→ Gotu kola (page 93)

→ Holy basil/tulsi (page 86)

→ Licorice (page 192)

→ Schisandra

When taken daily, and with consideration to diet and lifestyle, adaptogens provide general resiliency and a modulating effect. They support the body's resistance to all kinds of stressors—biological, chemical, and physical—by modulating the production of stress-related neurotransmitters and hormones. This is because adaptogenic herbs affect the way our stress response and the hypothalamic-pituitary-adrenal (HPA) axis of the nervous and endocrine systems communicate. In addition, each adaptogenic herb has its own unique healing capabilities, so take some time to consider which ones fit your health needs best.

The adaptogenic herbs mentioned in this book are on the more balancing and calming end of the spectrum. They provide a less "buzzy" form of energy support, soothing anxiety while nourishing and normalizing a broad range of conditions. Note that these herbs aren't calming in the sense that they are going to make you feel sleepy or unmotivated; the form of energy they provide is less zippy and more gradual and sustained. The four plants highlighted in this chapter—gotu kola, ashwagandha, licorice, and holy basil/tusli—gently enliven and are my go-to adaptogenic herbs when someone is navigating chronic illness, stress, overwhelm, insomnia, trauma, brain fog, fatigue, depression, anxiety, or issues with memory. Though more stimulating adaptogens like American or Asian ginseng can be helpful when used thoughtfully, I've chosen to only discuss the calming adaptogens because they are extremely effective at regulating and revitalizing the body without pushing you further into a burnout state, which can sometimes occur with the more stimulating adaptogens.

A question to ask yourself when deciding which, if any, adaptogen you should work with is: What is motivating my work with this plant? In our overworked, stressed-out, production-driven world, the more stimulating adaptogens have gained popularity because we are determined to go, go, go! We want to do it all— override our tired bodies and find some secret elixir that will allow us to have energy for days. Alas, our bodies were not meant to go, go, go.

In fact, many people are in such a constant state of burnout, running on empty, that to simply give the body more stimulating herbs without making lifestyle and mindset adjustments can cause further fatigue and damage to one's health. Remember, what our bodies need first and foremost is nourishment in the form of whole foods, rest, laughter, clean water, nature, physical connection, and daily movement. It's important to check in with the pillars of self-care in chapter 2 (page 33) before you start working with adaptogens. If you are open to embracing the work that comes with a healthy, balanced life, these potent and respected adaptogens will work wonders at bringing a depleted body back into harmony, replenishing and healing your deep self, and awakening your vitality. Adaptogens do not replace this work, they enrich it.

Vitality and Mental Clarity

Vitality on Your Own Terms

Every living organism deserves health and vitality. To feel vital, or strong in oneself, is to experience a liveliness of spirit—to feel rested upon waking, confident in your ability to handle the tasks of the day, and open to possibilities. Often in healing traditions, vitality is regarded as having a strong life force. I often think of vitality as the difference between surviving and thriving. We can survive, moving through life exhausted and stressed, but are we thriving? Are we alive and vital, feeling passionate, rested, creative, and curious?

To sustain our life force over the long term, it must be nurtured by the world around us. Like so many aspects of health, our ability to experience vitality is both a personal journey and an indicator of the priorities of our society. If we can only experience health and vitality, safety and joy, because of our social standing, race, gender expression, or financial status, what does that say about our society?

The first step is to make sure you're staying connected to your own personal, evolving experience of vitality. Release the notion that you lack something and instead consider the abundance around you, the possibilities of exactly where you are. Contemplate what your life force needs to thrive. Our culture is a bit out of step with the practices required for vitality, so it can often feel like you're swimming against the current to do what's right for your body and your health. Because of this, achieving a relationship with your vital self will be a mix of personal commitments and collective shifts. This doesn't mean health and vitality are out of reach for you—just that you may have to change your lifestyle to accommodate more rest and less screen time, or get creative when you come up against some frustrating hurdles like finding good-quality produce.

LIFESTYLE

Although we each access vitality from a personal perspective and have varying needs, a few things are universal for us to thrive. On a physical level, we need nutrient-rich foods, rest, movement, and clean drinking water. On an emotional and spiritual level we crave connection, contemplation, pleasure, and creativity.

When shifting beyond mere survival mode and wanting to replenish your vital force, I recommend first making sure all your most basic needs are met. Review the pillars of self-care in chapter 2 and look into herbs and practices that can assist with healthy digestion in chapter 3. If you have regular bowel movements, stay hydrated with plenty of water, eat a whole-foods diet, and get enough sleep, then it's time to make a commitment to seeking out the emotional and spiritual components and become a disciple of the art of being vital, of thriving.

PRACTICE: A DINNER PARTY FOR VITALITY

Communal eating used to be much more commonplace. Nowadays, many of us live alone, eat out more, or share a house with roommates who are constantly in and out. Sharing a meal—from planning and preparation to eating—has been proven to improve one's health. Shared meals support us in eating more nutritious foods and less junk food and having consistent mealtimes with intimacy and connection (with both ingredients and friends), empowerment from cooking your own meal, pleasure, intention, better dietary choices, and healthy digestion, all wrapped up in a dinner party.

Come up with a theme. If you're trying to support yourself with healthier eating, weave that into the mix. Center the meal around a certain in-season herb, a region of the world, or a cooking technique you want to experiment with. If you are trying to stay away from certain foods like gluten, dairy, sugar, or alcohol, make this known so your friends can support you in your diet and lifestyle commitments.

You can do this potluck style, asking that everyone come with a dish, or my favorite, invite the crew over to help cook, dividing tasks and sharing in drinks (herbal cocktails, anyone?) and conversation while everything is being prepared.

HERBS AND FLOWER ESSENCES

When working with herbal medicine to bring about and sustain vitality, start with nutritives. Nutritive herbs are vitamin- and mineral-rich sources of nutrition, as well as gentle and safe for everyone. Nettle and oat are two of my favorites. If you're new to working with herbs, these are a great introduction, as they are commercially available, easy to find, and well-suited for infusions, making them a great low-cost option.

If you want to work with flower essences to support vitality, start with nasturtium and oak. Nasturtium aids in improving vitality by rooting you in your body and calming that buzzy, frantic feeling of excessive mental energy. Oak fortifies personal integrity so that we can know our limits and ask for what we need.

Stinging Nettle (*Urtica dioica*)

PARTS USED leaf

ENERGETICS drying

When vibrant health and vitality are your aim, you can look no further than this often-dismissed weed. Beloved by herbalists far and wide, nettle has a long history as a nutritive herb and wild food source wherever it is abundant. Growing in the spring, nettle is commonly found in patches growing along flowing creeks. Nettle supports the immune, digestive, endocrine, nervous, urinary, and circulatory systems, making it a superior herb for the whole body. A spring tonic and rejuvenator, nettle is high in vitamins and minerals, including vitamins A, B complex, and C, along with iron, calcium, zinc, potassium, and magnesium. All those vitamins and minerals fortify healthy skin, bones, blood, nails, and hair and help drain or detoxify the body of toxins or excess fluids, which can be especially helpful in cases of gout, rheumatism, or edema. Nettle tincture can also assist in allergies as it regulates the inflammatory and histamine responses.

Due to its high levels of iron and magnesium, nettle is an especially nourishing tonic herb for the menstrual cycle. Try drinking a quart of nettle infusion every day and you'll notice your PMS symptoms and menstrual cramps decreasing over time. Generally, nettle will be supportive for anyone who feels lethargic or weak from anemia or chronic illness or has recurring muscle cramps due to poor nutrient absorption.

The best preparation for ingesting vitamins and minerals from an herb is a hot infusion left to steep for a minimum of an hour, though overnight is preferred.

WORD TO THE WISE Unlike the afternoon crash that's common when consuming coffee or energy drinks, nettle energizes while allowing you to feel grounded in your power throughout the day. Nettle gives a feeling of self-assuredness and inner strength; traditionally it was thought to offer protection. For a week, try replacing your coffee habit with nettle tea and try sipping the Restorative Overnight Nettle Infusion (page 83) throughout the day.

SUGGESTED PREPARATIONS hot overnight infusion, nettle pesto, syrup, tincture

FAVORITE PLANT PAIRINGS oatstraw, holy basil/tulsi

Restorative Overnight Nettle Infusion

Nettle, with its deep emerald color and earthy flavor, was one of the first herbs I fell in love with as a budding herbalist, and I hope you do too! Incorporating nettle into your daily routine can be a serious game-changer as you begin to benefit from the vitamins and minerals this beloved plant offers.

MAKES 4 CUPS

4 heaping tablespoons nettle leaf, cut and sifted

To make this restorative nettle infusion, add 4 tablespoons of dried nettle leaf (or a handful of fresh leaves) to a quart jar or French press. Bring water to a boil and pour over the herb the cover. Allow to steep overnight on the kitchen counter or keep in the fridge. Strain and reheat if desired or drink chilled.

Ashwagandha (*Withania somnifera*)

PARTS USED root

ENERGETICS slightly warming

A beloved plant in the Ayurvedic tradition, ashwagandha is an adaptogen that has been used for thousands of years for when one's vigor and zest for life is depleted due to chronic illness or stress. The root of this small, woody shrub offers the body a chance to gently restore vitality and energy by switching us from a strung-out, wired-and-tired energy to a more grounded, steady flow of energy. It is a deeply nourishing and strengthening tonic herb that enhances our ability to shift unhealthy patterns relating to self-worth and productivity. Many of us are stuck in a burnout mindset, limiting our ability to sink into rest and pleasure for the sake of getting things done. Our mind spins with the tasks of the day, and no matter how much our body craves rest, we can't seem to stop doing. Taken daily, ashwagandha encourages us to slow down and favor intentional action, rest, and pleasure over hurried productivity fueled by stimulants and workaholic tendencies.

Long-term use of ashwagandha tones the nervous, endocrine, and immune systems, making this warming, moistening plant ideal for those who struggle with insomnia, adrenal exhaustion, sexual dysfunction, chronic stress, or chronic immune conditions that benefit from an immune-modulating affect.

WORD TO THE WISE Ashwagandha's species name, *somnifera*, means "sleep-inducing," and this gentle sedative is favored in formulas when a person has trouble staying asleep (as opposed to getting to sleep), often waking up at the same early morning hour night after night. A subtle sedative, ashwagandha comes to the aid of insomnia sufferers, offering deep and dreamless sleep when taken long-term as part of a sleep ritual. For this, take a tincture of ashwagandha twice daily, and enjoy a cup of Ashwagandha Golden Milk (page 85) in the hour leading up to your bedtime.

SUGGESTED PREPARATIONS decoction, tincture, honey, ghee

FAVORITE PLANT PAIRINGS milky oat, holy basil/tulsi, passionflower

Ashwagandha Golden Milk

With a mix of warming and aromatic spices—grounding ashwagandha, steadying holy basil/tulsi, calming chamomile, and liver-loving dandelion root—this bold blend will steady and soothe. Have a cup as a warm after-dinner beverage to aid in digestion while setting the intention for a restful night's sleep.

MAKES 4 CUPS

1 tablespoon ashwagandha
1 tablespoon dandelion root
1 tablespoon holy basil/tulsi
2 teaspoons chamomile
1 teaspoon licorice
1 teaspoon ground turmeric
Pinch of black pepper

OPTIONAL: rose petals, vanilla bean, a cinnamon stick, and herbal honey
NOTE: All herbs should be cut and sifted.

To create the blend, add all the ingredients to a pint jar, put the lid on, and shake to combine. Label the jar with the blend title, ingredients, and the date you made it. Store it out of direct sunlight and it will keep for 8–12 months.

When ready to drink, use 1 tablespoon of the blend for every 8 ounces of water, milk, or milk alternative. For 1 serving, add 1 tablespoon to a reusable tea strainer. Alternatively, you can add ingredients to a small pot to brew up to 32 ounces. Bring liquid of choice to a gentle simmer for 5–10 minutes. Turn off the heat and allow to steep with the lid on for a minimum of 5 minutes.

Holy Basil/Tulsi (*Ocimum tenuiflorum*)

PARTS USED leaf and flower

ENERGETICS warming, drying

Holy basil, also known as *tulsi*, is considered the holiest of plants in India, where it has been used in Ayurveda for thousands of years. A fragrant member of the mint family and a close relative to the culinary basil (*Ocimum basilicum*) that we are more familiar with in the West, this adaptogen strengthens vitality and increases our adaptability to long-term and everyday stressors. Believed to be the earthly incarnation of the divine, holy basil is a transformative herb, helping us shift how we relate to life's ups and downs on a foundational level, strengthening our resilience and increasing joy.

If you are going through a time of uncertainty due to a life transition or unexpected news—a move, change of career, breakup, illness, death—and you wish you could just hit the pause button on life's demands and take care of yourself, holy basil is an excellent ally. This adaptogen clears the cobwebs from your mind and promotes mental clarity so you can still show up for your responsibilities.

On the physical level, holy basil protects the heart, lowers blood pressure, and stabilizes blood sugar. It can be used as an antimicrobial, supporting wound healing when used topically or in the case of herpes and shingles when taken internally. It reduces excessive immune response for those with chronic allergies and asthma, especially when asthma is triggered by stress. In general, it has a balancing effect on the immune system as a whole. As with most mint family plants, holy basil improves digestion and is an ideal medicine for the winter blues, when in low spirits, and when you have sluggish digestion due to holiday indulgences and overeating.

WORD TO THE WISE Holy basil is one of the easier adaptogens to grow in your garden, where it thrives much like culinary basil. A sunny spot, warm weather, and regular watering, and you'll have plenty to go around.

SUGGESTED PREPARATIONS tea, oxymel, tincture

FAVORITE PLANT PAIRINGS rose, nettle, oat, lemon balm

Sacred Spark Infusion

If you'd like to give up coffee without saying goodbye to caffeine altogether, try this infusion. With the stimulating blend of aromatic herbs like ginger, damiana, and rosemary; the nourishing qualities of nettle and holy basil that build up tired nerves; and antioxidant-rich green tea, you will find yourself happily grabbing for this every morning.

MAKES 4 CUPS

2 tablespoons nettle leaf

1 tablespoon holy basil/tulsi

1 tablespoon damiana

2 teaspoons green tea or yerba mate

1 teaspoon fresh or dried ginger

1 teaspoon fresh or dried rosemary

NOTE: All herbs should be cut and sifted.

To make the blend, add all the ingredients to a small jar, put the lid on, and shake thoroughly to combine. Label the jar with the blend title, ingredients, and the date you made it. Store the blend out of direct sunlight and it will keep for 8–12 months.

When ready to drink, use 1 tablespoon of the blend for every 8 ounces of water. For 1 serving, add 1 tablespoon to a reusable tea strainer. Alternatively, you can add the tea blend to a glass jar or French press and brew up to 32 ounces. Bring water to a boil and pour it over the blend and allow to steep for a minimum of 15 minutes. Enjoy hot or refrigerate and enjoy chilled.

Mental Clarity, Memory, and Focus

We all can relate to that feeling of walking into a room only to completely forget what brought us there in the first place. Forgetfulness, lack of focus or attention, and brain fog can be serious frustrations as we navigate our days. The good news is that herbs, along with diet and lifestyle changes, can do wonders to support brain health and target any underlying issues you're dealing with.

LIFESTYLE

Daily exercise can play a huge role in keeping your mind in tip-top shape. Community engagement, trying new things, time in nature, reading, mental games, plenty of time to relax, and a good night's sleep are also critical.

Consider journaling, meditating (which has been scientifically proven to support cognition and focus), working on being present with the tasks and people in front of you (instead of multitasking and doing too much at once), and not overloading your schedule. An overly busy, stressful lifestyle is going to make focus and calm difficult. Try to acknowledge your own personal threshold and set boundaries for what you can accomplish each week while maintaining healthy eating and rest.

PRACTICE: MINDFUL PHONE USE

Have you ever wondered if the smartphones and tablets so many of us are glued to all the time are messing with our ability to retain information, think clearly, and focus? Like anything else, there are healthy ways to interact with technology and unhealthy ways. If you're struggling with memory and focus, if you can't seem to overcome your brain fog, mental fatigue, anxiety, or forgetfulness, then consider how, when, and why you use your phone.

It's important to acknowledge that these devices and the ways we use them influence how the brain functions. The truth is, our devices affect both short- and long-term memory, disrupting our ability to retain information and leaving little mental space for new memories. Our capacity to take in and recall new information is called the *working memory*, and it's pretty limited and easily overloaded. When it gets overloaded, we experience mental fatigue and difficulty concentrating.

The truth is, our devices affect both
short- and long-term memory, disrupting our
ability to retain information and leaving little
mental space for new memories.

Due in part to the omnipresence of smartphones, we've come to expect a constant, fast stream of quickly evolving information. Constantly scrolling through images, e-mails, articles, posts, and status updates keeps our minds bouncing from one thing to the next. This lack of sustained concentration on one thing, along with absentminded reliance on apps and social media, can send us down the slippery slope of mental overload, compassion fatigue, anxiety, lack of focus, forgetfulness, and brain fog.

HERBS AND FLOWER ESSENCES

Most herbs recommended for mental clarity and focus do so by awakening your senses, improving circulation and mood, supporting the nervous system, and fighting inflammation. Aromatic mint family plants like basil, lemon balm, peppermint, rosemary, sage, and spearmint are great because of their high volatile oil content. Plus, they are easy to grow whether you have a large garden plot or a small windowsill; they are versatile, affordable, and widely available. With any of these herbs, the scent alone can clear a foggy headspace, improve memory, and enliven mood. You don't even have to pick these plants to benefit from them; simply rub your hands through a patch of rosemary or mint, bring your hands to your face, and inhale deeply.

In addition, black pepper, calamus, garlic, ginger, gingko, gotu kola, green tea, holy basil/tulsi, and lion's mane all promote healthy brain function by supporting circulation and nerve health, stimulating mental cognition, and soothing inflammation. Common issues underlying brain fog, forgetfulness, dementia, and attention issues include stress, systemic inflammation, and poor gut health, so incorporating herbs like calendula, damiana, nettle, oatstraw, skullcap, and wood betony can help.

If you want to work with flower essences to support memory and focus, try lemon blossom and broom to start. Lemon blossom is an uplifting and lighthearted essence, excellent if making decisions overwhelms you or if you have difficulty feeling clearheaded in the face of many options. Broom supports you in mental clarity and concentration, helping to keep your mind flexible and adaptable while supporting your capacity to learn, remember, and recall information.

Rosemary (*Rosmarinus officinalis*)

PARTS USED leaf

ENERGETICS warming, drying

Very few plants greet us as heartily as fragrant rosemary. A favorite aromatic culinary and garden herb, rosemary has longstanding use in Mediterranean and European herbal traditions. In European folklore, rosemary is a plant of remembrance. We can carry this traditional use forward, working with rosemary in moments of grief as we process loss and strike a balance between remembering and releasing those we hold dear. Rosemary grounds us as we open ourselves to difficult feelings.

Today, rosemary is best known as a tonic for the nervous system, strengthening memory and focus. Interestingly, Greek scholars were known to wear a garland of rosemary on their heads to help with memory during examinations. During exams week, try keeping a sprig of rosemary in your pocket or take it as a tea, tincture, or oxymel while you study. An ally for those with poor circulation who tend to feel chilled and have sluggish digestion, rosemary is a stimulating herb that will bring warmth and movement to both systems and is especially beneficial for the elderly. If indigestion, gas, or bloating are common complaints, cook with rosemary often or create an after-meal ritual with this plant. Dried or fresh rosemary is a lovely addition to a ritual bath or foot soak. Combined with nettle as an infusion, it's also an effective hair rinse for stimulating follicle health. At the first sign of allergies or an upper respiratory complaint, prepare an herbal steam (page 175) by simmering a pot of water with fresh or dried rosemary and breathe in the healing aromatics.

Rely on rosemary, a respected antimicrobial, internally or externally for all manner of colds and infections. Whether you need protection from germs or bad vibes, versatile rosemary can help.

WORD TO THE WISE Traditionally, rosemary was used as an herb of protection, hung above doorways or planted outside the home to ward off evil spirits. It was used in the infamous Four Thieves blend that kept grave robbers untouched by infection while robbing victims during the plague.

SUGGESTED PREPARATIONS honey, steam, oxymel or vinegar, bath, hot infusion, flower essence

FAVORITE PLANT PAIRINGS wood betony, damiana, gotu kola, holy basil/tulsi, ginger

Grounded Focus Tincture

This tincture is a deeply supportive blend that encourages calm while feeding your nerves, strengthening your nervous system, and enhancing overall cognition, clarity of mind, and focus.

MAKES 4-OUNCE (120 ML) BOTTLE

40 milliliters lion's mane alcohol extract

25 milliliters gotu kola alcohol extract

20 milliliters rosemary alcohol extract

20 milliliters milky oat alcohol extract

15 milliliters wood betony alcohol extract

See page 235 for instructions on making a tincture.

Take 1–2 dropperfuls twice daily for an extended period (minimum 4–6 weeks) to help with overall cognition, nervous-system support, and focus. In a pinch, for more acute situations, take 1–2 dropperfuls whenever mental fatigue and stress inhibit your ability to focus. This tincture can be added to a few inches of drinking water, added to a smoothie or juice, or put directly in the mouth.

Brain Tonic Tincture

When you are feeling mentally fatigued and out of it, these herbs will help tone and encourage brain health, improve cerebral circulation, nourish nerves, steady the mind, and keep you focused and alert without a buzzy feeling or overstimulation. Reach for this tincture anytime you want to enhance your mental capabilities.

MAKES 2-OUNCE (60 ML) BOTTLE

20 milliliters gotu kola alcohol extract
20 milliliters gingko alcohol extract
10 milliliters milky oat alcohol extract
10 milliliters rosemary alcohol extract

See page 235 for instructions on making a tincture.

Take 1–2 dropperfuls twice daily for an extended period (minimum 4–6 weeks) to help with brain fog, mental fatigue, nervousness, or overwhelm. For more acute situations, take 1–2 dropperfuls whenever you want to feel energized and clearheaded. This tincture can be added to a few inches of drinking water, added to a smoothie or juice, or put directly in the mouth.

Gotu Kola (*Centella asiatica*)

PARTS USED leaf

ENERGETICS cooling, drying

We all experience forgetfulness from time to time, but when our days are marked by confusion, misplaced belongings, and brain fog, it might be time to contemplate how we're supporting our brain health. Native to tropical and subtropical regions of Asia, Africa, and the Americas, gotu kola, commonly known as pennywort, is a botanical ally most relied on for its effects on memory and focus. Studies show that gotu kola promotes cerebral circulation, which in turn helps with focus, concentration, and memory while it revitalizes the nerves and brain cells. A deeply restoring and balancing nervous-system tonic, gotu kola improves circulation and builds mental resiliency with consistent use.

Used successfully in the treatment of Alzheimer's, gotu kola creates subtle shifts in our ability to remember information. Used for thousands of years in Indonesia, India, and China, gotu kola is both a food and a medicine, showing up fresh in salads and potent medicinal formulas alike.

WORD TO THE WISE Beyond its brain-boosting abilities, gotu kola is often used to reduce scarring; quicken healing time for wounds, burns, and scrapes; and is an excellent addition to face and skin oils, especially if you have acne scars.

SUGGESTED PREPARATIONS salads, hot infusions, body oil, tincture

FAVORITE PLANT PAIRINGS rosemary, holy basil/tulsi, reishi, calendula, gingko

Gotu Kola Rose Facial Oil

This oil utilizes gotu kola and calendula, two herbs that can't be beat when it comes to health and healing inside and out. Since our skin is our largest organ of absorption, the kind of body-care products we rely on should be free of synthetic fragrance and harmful additives. Prized for its ability to reduce redness, encourage circulation, and increase the synthesis of collagen, gotu kola should be a mainstay in both your beauty and brain-health routines.

MAKES 8-OUNCE JAR

3 tablespoons gotu kola
2 tablespoons calendula
1 tablespoon rose
1 cup carrier oil(s) of choice

NOTE: All herbs should be cut and sifted.

See page 237 for instructions on making herbal oil.

To use, add a few drops to the tips of your fingers and massage on clean skin, prioritizing areas on your face where dry skin, redness, or acne scars are an issue. This oil can be used as an all-over moisturizing daily facial oil or for a scar-minimizing, skin-rejuvenating spot treatment in your skin-care routine.

NOTE: Some of my favorite carrier oils are organic, cold-pressed, unrefined almond, apricot kernel, argan, borage seed, jojoba, rose hips, sea buckthorn, and sunflower. Pick one or combine several.

Brain-Boosting Infusion

Looking to clear the cobwebs, enhance circulation, invigorate the senses, and lift your mood? Look no further than this Brain-Boosting Infusion, a favorite when exhaustion and stress have given way to brain fog, lack of focus, and low spirits. This can also be enjoyed when you are under the weather and in a haze.

MAKES 4 CUPS

2 tablespoons gotu kola
1 tablespoon holy basil/tulsi
1 tablespoon lemon balm
1 tablespoon fresh ginger

NOTE: All herbs should be cut and sifted.

To make the blend, add all the ingredients to a small jar, put the lid on, and shake thoroughly to combine. Label the jar with the blend title, ingredients, and the date you made it. Store the blend out of direct sunlight and it will keep for 8–12 months.

To prepare this Brain-Boosting Infusion, use 1 heaping tablespoon of the blend for every 8 ounces of water. For a single serving, add 1 tablespoon to a reusable tea strainer. Alternatively, you can add the blend to a glass jar or French press and brew up to 32 ounces. Bring water to a boil and pour it over the blend and allow to steep for a minimum of 15 minutes. Enjoy hot or refrigerate and enjoy chilled.

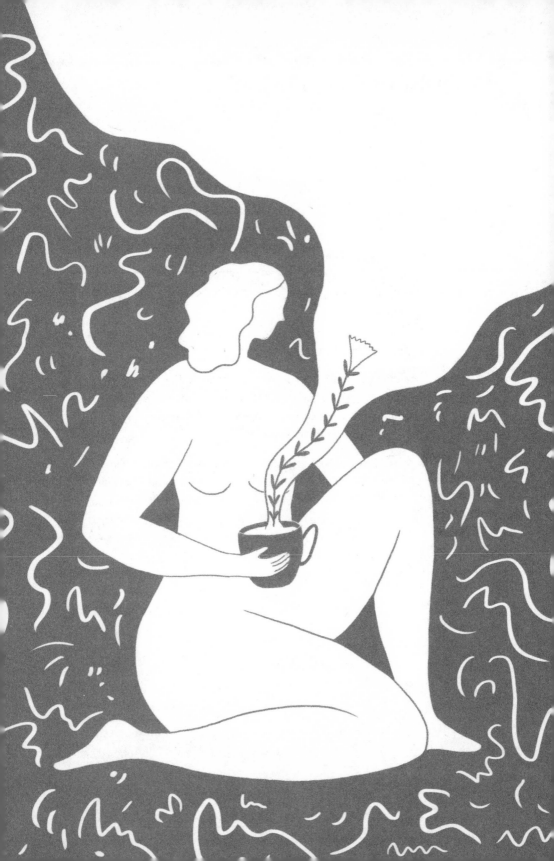

Navigating Stress and Anxiety

5

WHEN WE FEEL STRESSED OR ANXIOUS, it becomes increasingly difficult to prioritize self-care. As our awareness is pulled in a million different directions, we forsake all the thoughtful actions we do to keep feeling our best. So how exactly do we navigate stress and anxiety with self-care?

For starters, you let go of any notion of perfection and offer yourself a heaping dose of compassion. Everyone has a tough time showing up for themselves when life gets cluttered and stressful, when we're anxious or upset. You're a human doing the best you can in a messy world.

This is the complexity of being alive at a time when we want to do it all, feel as though we should be able to, and live in a culture that makes us feel inadequate if we can't keep up. Talk about stress and anxiety! More importantly, so much of our current world is oppressive, imbalanced, and unsustainable. Over the years, my greatest lesson for mental health has been to recognize and remember that the society we live in is sick, making personal health and self-care even more difficult. Stress and anxiety are actually healthy responses when we try to keep up with or fit into systems that are toxic and dysfunctional. It takes a lot of trial and error, plenty of dedication to self-love and self-preservation, and the help of our favorite herbal allies and chosen support systems to keep us on track. All you can do is the best you can with what you've got.

Stress

A stressor is anything that puts a demand on us, good or bad. Stress is a whole-body process, and stressors come in many physiological and psychological forms, from the pain of a broken heart to the pain of a cut on your finger. When every-day stress becomes routine, we experience chronic stress—consistent, low-level stress day in and day out. This happens when our healthy stress response is overly activated and never has time to come back into balance. It's the stress of having too much on your plate for an extended period of time—hating your job for years, consistently eating a poor diet, dealing with daily microaggressions due to your race, age, mental health, gender expression, or sexual orientation. All of these have the potential to make us feel stressed-out, depleted, and unable to calmly navigate our days.

> Stress is not the enemy;
> it is a teacher and a way our body tells us
> we are overloaded and need to pause.

The good news is that experiencing this kind of pressure gives us an oppor-tunity to show up by making appropriate lifestyle changes, fighting for change in our communities and in the world, and being honest about what we're willing and able to take on. In addition, working with herbs can offer significant support. It's crucial that we learn to identify stressors and experience stress in a healthy man-ner. Stress is not the enemy; it is a teacher and a way our body tells us we are over-loaded and need to pause.

Although it's no fun to be stressed-out, this natural response is a sophisti-cated function that evolved to keep us out of harm's way. The thing is, the human body hasn't evolved to the rapidly changing demands of the modern world. Try to identify what aspects of your life create unnecessary stress and ask yourself how you can create a healthier response to moments when you feel overwhelmed. Can you remove the stressor, or do you need to build supportive practices that allow you to thrive regardless? What is the root cause of this stress? Does it require personal inquiry, a conversation with a loved one, community involve-ment, structural or societal shifts? What self-care practices can aid you this very moment so you can continue?

Side Effects of Stress

Here are some ways stress can affect our health:

→ Depression and anxiety

→ Brain fog and memory issues

→ Sleep disruption and insomnia

→ Skin issues

→ Feeling fatigued, or what I call "wired and tired"

→ Suppressed immune function, which can lead to higher rates of disease and poor wound healing

→ Increased production of certain inflammatory white blood cells

→ Poor metabolism, including elevated levels of cortisol and blood sugar, which can lead to diabetes and weight gain

→ Decreased libido and impaired generative health and function

→ Increased inflammation and increased risk of autoimmune disorders and inflammation-related diseases

→ Aggravation of longstanding conditions such as chronic allergies, asthma, arthritis, and irritable bowel syndrome

→ Slow digestion, indigestion, poor elimination, poor nutrient absorption, gas, and bloating

→ Diminished cardiovascular health, impaired circulation, high blood pressure, and high cholesterol levels

LIFESTYLE

Stress is an inescapable part of life and a fundamental part of being alive. So how we respond and relate to stress can make all the difference in the world. After all, modern life is full of stressors, making the purpose of self-care twofold. First, we must establish daily practices that build resiliency for all life throws at us. This will help us meet the stress of unforeseen challenges and new opportunities with flexibility and self-assuredness. Second, we must create the time to do practices that honor us whenever we are tired, sick, or overloaded, when we've had enough and life feels like too much.

To begin, a healthy diet is critical to nervous-system function and stress response. Start by getting plenty of omega-3 fatty acids, which can be found in wild-caught fish like herring and salmon, as well as in chia seeds, flax, hemp, and seaweeds. Make sure you're eating foods and herbs rich in vitamins such as vitamin D and B complex, and minerals like calcium, magnesium, and zinc, which can all be found in seaweeds like kelp or nori, alfalfa, chickweed, dandelion leaf and root, dark leafy greens, horsetail, nettle, and oatstraw.

PRACTICE: BE OF SERVICE TO YOUR BODY

How often does your body tell you what it needs but you ignore it or feel burdened by it? What about when you feel tired in the evening but push yourself to stay up for another few hours because "it's not bedtime yet" or because your friends are pressuring you to come out? Or at the first signs of illness, when all your body wants is to stay warm and rest, you pride yourself on sucking it up and pushing through?

It's important to think in terms of working in service of our bodies and listening to what stressors tell us. To listen to the signals your body is sending, you must slow down. Think about how difficult it can be to really listen to what someone is saying when you're being mentally pulled in a million different directions. You might nod in agreement, but are you really listening? Chances are, you're not. The same is true for your body. You have to make an effort to pause, pay attention, and listen to what your body is telling you, just as you would when you really want to hear what someone is saying.

To establish this relationship with your body, try to expand your awareness beyond your mind. After all, your entire body is taking in information, and to listen you have to quiet your overactive thoughts. Do something nice for your body—put on your favorite perfume, trust your gut, take a bath, go for a run, dance, anoint yourself with herbal oils, lie in the grass, cuddle, give yourself a massage, stretch.

If you've experienced trauma, chronic illness, or years of chronic stress and fatigue, you may require the support of a professional health-care provider or therapist to learn how to get in touch with your body. In fact, everyone can benefit from some outside support. Depending on your needs, you can get this from a Somatic Experiencing practitioner, a trauma-informed clinical herbalist, a massage or craniosacral therapist, an integrative or holistic psychiatrist, an acupuncturist, a mindfulness meditation class, or a breathwork session.

Forest Bathing

When we don't engage in unstructured time to play and explore in nature, stress, anxiety, depression, and attention-deficit issues escalate. Our body and mind crave time outdoors, and forest bathing, a term coined by the Forestry Agency of Japan in the early 1980s, is one way to nurture our innate wild nature. Forest bathing has become a cornerstone of Japanese preventative health care. The premise is quite simple. For starters, it has nothing to do with taking a bath in a forest (though that does sound wonderfully revitalizing!). It's more that you are taking in the atmosphere of a forest by walking, meditating, exercising, playing, or just existing among the flora, fauna, fresh air, and sunlight.

Apparently, doing these kinds of activities in nature offers even more physical and emotional benefits than doing them at home or in a gym. Leave your technology (yes, your phone!) in the car and sit or wander among the trees and plants. Even after just a few moments you'll notice how much more relaxed and present you feel.

HERBS AND FLOWER ESSENCES

To help keep you calm, grounded, and feeling your best, try drinking a daily nourishing infusion with herbs like:

- → Chamomile
- → Damiana
- → Dandelion root
- → Hawthorn
- → Holy basil/tulsi
- → Lemon balm

- → Nettle
- → Oat
- → Reishi
- → Rose
- → Skullcap
- → Wood betony

Consistent consumption of these herbs can nourish and strengthen the body as well as support you through a range of stress-induced issues such as fatigue and mental exhaustion, digestive distress, chronic illness flare-ups, headaches, hypertension, depression, anxiety, and the jitters.

> It's important to think in terms of working in service
> of our bodies and listening to what stressors tell us.

If you want to work with flower essences to support yourself in dealing with stress, try self-heal and yarrow to start. Self-heal (*Prunella vulgaris*), also known as "heal-all," is an easy-to-grow plant in the mint family with sweet purple flowers. When taken as an essence it helps us prioritize our health needs. Self-heal nudges us gently toward the pillars of self-care (see chapter 2), because when we're stressed, we need to commit to our foundational needs more than ever. Yarrow is another indispensable ally when you are stressed and overloaded but have trouble saying no. If you often experience stress because you put too much on your plate or bend over backward to help everyone when you're already depleted, it's time to learn boundaries, and yarrow is great for that.

Oat (*Avena sativa*)

PARTS USED milky seed, oatstraw

ENERGETICS neutral

Oat is among the best nutrient-rich tonic herbs for the nervous system. Oat is a nutritive herb for anxiety and fatigue and feeds the nervous system especially when under stress or due to a lifestyle of overwork. It can be especially helpful if you are prone to irritability, tension headaches, or forgetfulness regarding your basic needs when your plate is full.

Oat is an excellent source of magnesium, which relaxes tight muscles and cramping. Try drinking a quart of oatstraw infusion throughout the day when tense muscles or menstrual cramps become an issue.

A tincture of milky oat, which is harvested when the seeds produce a milky substance when squeezed, reinforces strong nerve endings, acting as a buffer between us and the world. If you are more introverted and find being social a little taxing or flat-out overwhelming, oatstraw infusion or milky oat tincture before and after social events can reinforce and soothe an overexcited nervous system. Oat can also be an excellent ally when you find yourself trying to quit an addictive habit like smoking or drinking. Combine with licorice, passionflower, and skullcap for support when quitting an addictive habit.

WORD TO THE WISE Oatmeal, steel-cut oats, oatstraw, and milky oat all come from the same plant, *Avena sativa*. Each are harvested at different times and go through different amounts of processing. Oatmeal and steel-cut oats are often stored and processed in commercial facilities alongside wheat, barley, or rye, causing cross-contamination and the need for oats to be labeled "gluten-free." Otherwise, oats do not contain gluten, so if you're using them medicinally, whether you're purchasing a milky oat tincture or oatstraw from a medicinal herb farm (medicinal herb farms rarely, if ever, grow crops like wheat, barley, and rye) or a small-scale medicine-maker, you don't have to worry about cross-contamination. That said, you're welcome to ask farmers and medicine-makers questions, and you should always pay attention to the subtle shifts and signs your body gives you when you begin to work with a new plant ally. If something feels off, trust that feeling and chat with an herbalist or health-care provider.

FAVORITE PREPARATIONS oatstraw hot infusion, herbal bath, milky oat tincture

SUGGESTED PLANT PAIRINGS nettle, ashwagandha, damiana, skullcap

Milky Oat, Ashwagandha, and Rose Tincture

This trio is an all-time favorite that I rarely go without. A subtle buffer from life's hardships, milky oat, rose, and ashwagandha combine to encourage a calm and composed feeling.

MAKES 2-OUNCE (60 ML) BOTTLE

25 milliliters milky oat alcohol extract

20 milliliters ashwagandha alcohol extract

15 milliliters rose alcohol extract

See page 235 for instructions on making a tincture.

Take 1–2 dropperfuls twice daily for an extended period—minimum 4–6 weeks—to help with stress, anxiety, sleeplessness, worry, fatigue, agitation, anger, or overwhelm. This tincture can be added to a few inches of drinking water, added to a smoothie or juice, or put directly in mouth.

Stress Less Infusion

The name says it all! This infusion should be in the drinking water! Stress Less Infusion is your daily tea for nervous-system nourishment. With herbs that are vitamin and mineral powerhouses, Stress Less helps build you up while offering support in case of stress, worry, overwhelm, exhaustion, mental fatigue, and more.

MAKES 4 CUPS

> 2 tablespoons oatstraw
> 2 tablespoons lemon balm
> 1 tablespoon nettle
> 2 teaspoons holy basil/tulsi
> 2 teaspoons alfalfa

NOTE: All herbs should be cut and sifted.

To make the blend, add all ingredients to a small jar, put the lid on, and shake thoroughly to combine. Label the jar with the blend title, ingredients, and the date you made it. Store the blend out of direct sunlight and it will keep for 8–12 months.

When ready to drink Stress Less Infusion, use 1 heaping tablespoon of the blend for every 8 ounces of water. For a single serving, add 1 tablespoon of the blend to a reusable tea strainer. Alternatively, you can add the blend to a glass jar or French press and brew up to 32 ounces. Bring water to a boil and pour it over the blend and allow it to steep for a minimum of 15 minutes. Even better, try steeping overnight. Enjoy hot or refrigerate and enjoy chilled.

Trust Your Ease Syrup

A delicious blend of calming, balancing, uplifting, and aromatic herbs, Trust Your Ease relaxes the body and quiets the mind, plus it tastes great!

MAKES 3 CUPS

> 4 cups water
> 3 tablespoons oatstraw
> 2 tablespoons lemon balm
> 2 tablespoons rose hips
> 1 tablespoon holy basil/tulsi
> 1 tablespoon orange peel
> 1 cup sweetener of choice—local raw honey or
> unrefined cane sugar usually works best

See page 227 for instructions on making a syrup.

Take up to a tablespoon of syrup twice daily to support yourself through life's stresses. Syrup can be added to sparkling or filtered water or a cup of tea, mixed into a smoothie or breakfast oats, or taken straight into the mouth using a dropper bottle. When using a dropper bottle, 3–4 dropperfuls will equal about 1 teaspoon. Store syrup in the refrigerator and it will last for up to 6 months.

Anxiety

Anxiety is a state of apprehension, worry, or dread that can come on when we're experiencing something new or upsetting. These feelings may present as a general uneasiness or may be connected to specific stressors that you recognize over time, like large social gatherings or public speaking. Anxiety can also be large and overarching, a symptom of a world with grave injustice and ecological destruction or of societies modeled for profit and production instead of fulfillment and pleasure. When you are overworked and exhausted, your frayed nervous system can become reactive and anxious.

Like any other sensation we experience, anxiety can be viewed as a message from your body. Much like stress, experiencing occasional anxiety or jitters is a completely natural, healthy response that serves a purpose. This is why it's important to incorporate dietary, lifestyle, and herbal practices into how you work with your anxiety instead of dismissing it or trying to cover it up.

If your anxiety is occasional and mild, allow it to work as a teacher in your life. Does it occur in certain social situations? After a week of poor sleep or eating? Whenever you eat a certain food or hang out with a certain person? During a certain time in your menstrual cycle? Or is it due to social or environmental unrest in your community or around the world? This is a subtle conversation your body is trying to have with you. Listen and take note. Work with herbs to build up your fatigued nervous system so it can better buffer you from stress and help you get the rest you require. You can also get involved in social activism causes that speak to you or donate to organizations that you care about.

If your anxiety is inhibiting you from enjoying life, take comfort in knowing that herbs, diet, and lifestyle shifts can support you. You can also benefit from working with a professional who can help map out your health needs and recommend a personalized protocol. In my experience, trying to work through health stuff by yourself can feel overwhelming and can bring on worry. There is definitely support beyond this book out there for you, but in the meantime, brew a cup of chamomile, lemon balm, and passionflower tea or take a dropperful of kava tincture, and try one of the following practices.

LIFESTYLE

Experiencing anxiety? Let's simplify.

→ Where are you doing too much, promising too much of yourself, overextending yourself?

→ What aspect of life and in what ways are you trying to control events or people?

→ Where in your body do you hold tension?

→ What are you afraid of and what's the worst that could happen? Are you getting ahead of yourself? Making assumptions?

→ When was the last time you ate a solid meal and drank a glass of water?

→ When was the last time you got a good night's sleep?

These are the questions I want you to ask yourself or even journal about, next time you are spinning out and anxious. When in doubt, practice breathwork (page 109), drink a glass of water, and get into your body (if it's safe to do so). Breathe into any tension you're holding in your body, relax your shoulders and the muscles in your face, and do some stretches. Rub your body down with an herbal oil. By touching your body—your arms, legs, feet, shoulders, neck, abdomen, wherever— you bring your focus back to your physical sensations and away from the buzzing thoughts in your mind.

In today's hustle and bustle, being fully embodied and grounded in yourself can be a real challenge. It's easy to get caught up replaying past upsets or worrying about the future. Many of us have experienced trauma or internalized messages of shame or hatred when it comes to our bodies, making our experiences of full embodiment all the more difficult. In addition, we are constantly inundated with stimuli, and in our commitment to staying informed, we live in our heads and run ourselves ragged. In this state we never fully relate to our bodies.

Grounding practices vary, but usually they engage the senses, focus on breath, and encourage us to be in touch with our body, both literally and figuratively, so we can fully engage in the here and now. Practices like self-massage with herbal oils, sipping an aromatic herbal tea blend, pausing to smell a flower, meditating, and even sitting under a tree for a few moments or standing barefoot in the grass can help to alleviate anxiety. These practices encourage a sense of rooted calm and focus and are versatile and uncomplicated ways to quiet the noise and come back to yourself.

Radical Remedies

Take off your shoes and plant your feet firmly on the ground, ask for a hug from someone you feel comfortable with, cuddle with your pet, prepare a cup of tea. Wiggle and shake it out, go on a run, jog or dance in place—anything to move out the anxious energy. You might look a little silly, but don't get caught up in what others think of you. What better time than now to prioritize your health and let go of how you're perceived—something you will never be able to control.

In addition, if you're prone to anxiety, worry, looping thoughts, and overwhelm, one of the best gifts you can give yourself is to limit or altogether avoid processed foods, especially sugary snacks and caffeinated, overly stimulating beverages. Replace these drinks with nerve-nourishing tonics and nutrient-rich tea blends like Restorative Overnight Nettle Infusion (page 83), Sacred Spark Infusion (page 87), or Stress Less Infusion (page 105).

PRACTICE: BREATHWORK

Breathwork is an active practice in which you focus your attention on your breath and connect with yourself. All you need to do to get started is to take a few deep breaths. When we come back to the breath, we quiet the mind and create space to settle into ourselves and the present moment. Sometimes just a few deep breaths can completely shift how we're experiencing stress, allowing us to make important decisions or assert boundaries, or even help us ground back into ourselves after experiencing anxiety or a panic attack.

One of my favorite breathing techniques, box breathing, is super simple. Get in a comfy position, either sitting or lying on the floor, though you can try this whenever—on an evening walk, while driving, and so on. If you're at home, you could burn some incense or prepare a cup of grounding ritual tea to sip afterward.

Close your eyes if you wish (not while driving, please!) and breathe in through your nose for four seconds, allowing your lungs to slowly fill with air. Hold the breath for four seconds. Then slowly exhale through your nose for four seconds, followed by another four seconds of holding. Repeat. Do this for a couple minutes or until you begin to feel calm and grounded.

HERBS AND FLOWER ESSENCES

When talking with folks about anxiety, worry, panic, and overwhelm, my first questions are: Where does the anxiety show up in your body? What are the physical sensations that accompany your anxiety? Does your heart race? Do you feel tightness in your chest? Do you notice tension in your shoulders? Get headaches? GI tract upset? These signals will help you narrow down which herbs will offer the most support.

Tinctures and flower essences are two of my favorite preparations for anxiety, as you can carry them discreetly and take immediately whenever they are needed without any fuss. When you take a tincture, commit to a moment to ground your mind and body. Simply put, grounding means coming back into your body fully. It means steering your awareness away from all the thoughts and worries swirling around in your head and touching base with your breath, the visceral sensations of your body, and the present moment.

Herbs that soothe anxiety by promoting grounding and calm include:

→ Blue vervain

→ Chamomile

→ Damiana

→ Garden sage

→ Hawthorn

→ Holy basil/tulsi

→ Kava

→ Lavender

→ Lemon balm

→ Motherwort

→ Passionflower

→ Rosemary

→ Wood betony

A Note on Dosing for Anxiety

Now that you're starting to understand that there are different ways you can work with herbs depending on the plant and the complaint, you'll also want to consider dosing. If you tend to experience anxiety, you might take a daily, tonic formula (page 25) of holy basil/tulsi, oat, rose, skullcap, and wood betony as a tea or tincture to nourish your nervous system long-term. But in a moment of anxiety or a panic attack—say, before a long flight, after running into an ex, or before public speaking—you'll want to reach for an acute formula (page 26). Tinctures can be taken in larger doses, are fast acting, and are easier to take on the go. Try herbs like kava, motherwort, passionflower, and skullcap for moments of anxiety.

The recommended dosing you see on most herbal tinctures at your local natural grocery store aren't personalized to your specific needs. When it comes to sleep disturbances or anxiety, for example, you may want to take larger doses. Let's say the recommended dosing on the bottle is 1–2 dropperfuls (30–60 drops). Start there and see how you feel. If you're still anxious or upset, you can dose much more, depending on your needs.

As a general rule, take between 1–4 dropperfuls (30–120 drops) every 5–15 minutes until you begin to settle and calm down. This is called *pulse dosing* and is also recommended when experiencing insomnia. If symptoms have settled but you continue to feel on edge, take 1–2 dropperfuls hourly. If you find yourself pulse dosing many times throughout the day for more than a week, seek out a better support system—reach out to friends or a trained herbalist, therapist, or health-care provider and shift to working with more tonic herbs.

Kava (*Piper methysticum*)

PARTS USED root

ENERGETICS warming, drying

A South Pacific ceremonial plant, kava (also known as kava kava) is a calming nervine that has been used traditionally for centuries, encouraging us to feel at peace and interact with others without worry. It is one of the most effective and safest relaxants in the plant kingdom, without any overly sedative effects. It acts as a mood elevator so that we can experience pleasure and intimacy with presence and clarity.

Kava has the ability to soothe tension in the body and is a lovely remedy when aches and tight muscles keep you from being fully present (try a kava massage oil). A generous ally to those fraught with anxiety, kava will chill out an overactive mind almost immediately. This plant medicine is ideal for those dealing with body insecurities, performance anxiety, or any issue where the mind loops negative thoughts.

WORD TO THE WISE Kava is a culturally significant herb with a small growing region—predominately Pacific Island nations that are at the forefront of the effects of global warming. Be conscientious about your use of kava for these reasons and consider if there are local or regional herbs you could be working with alternatively for anxiety and muscle tension.

SUGGESTED PREPARATIONS elixir, cold infusion, body oil

FAVORITE PLANT PAIRINGS damiana, rose, motherwort, passionflower

CAUTION This plant is not recommended for daily, long-term use, especially if you have liver damage.

Don't Panic! Acute Tincture

This can be a great formula for those preflight jitters, before a big presentation or public speaking engagement, or whatever might have you feeling anxious. Motherwort is a cool, nurturing hug of an herb and is excellent if your anxiety shows up in your chest with tightness, heaviness, or heart palpitations, while kava imparts an unabashed nod of confidence and calm self-assurance.

MAKES 2-OUNCE (60 ML) BOTTLE

20 milliliters kava alcohol extract
20 milliliters motherwort alcohol extract
20 milliliters passionflower alcohol extract

See page 235 for instructions on making a tincture.

Take 1–3 dropperfuls every 5–20 minutes, or until symptoms of anxiety, panic, or nervousness subside. This tincture can be added to a few inches of drinking water, added to a smoothie or juice, or put directly in the mouth. See "A Note on Dosing for Anxiety" (page 111) to better understand this dosing method and how to support yourself during acute moments of panic.

Motherwort (*Leonurus cardiaca*)

PARTS USED leaf

ENERGETICS cooling, drying

The Latin botanical name of motherwort, *Leonurus cardiaca*, means "lionhearted," which gives us an idea of the healing power of this mint family plant. There's nothing better than motherwort for when anxieties show up with heart palpitations and tightness in the chest. Motherwort temporarily lowers blood pressure and generally chills out an overactive nervous system so we can coolly tend to the tasks of the day.

Traditionally, motherwort was used during times of hormonal fluctuation, particularly during menstruation for PMS or menopausal complaints like hot flashes and night sweats. It also encourages blood flow and circulation, bringing on scanty, late, or irregular menstruation. As a bitter herb, motherwort improves digestion and supports the liver in the detoxification of excess hormones; it soothes cramps and muscle tension and spasms throughout the body.

Not only does this plant support our physical selves, but motherwort also comforts emotional distress and calms nervous irritability, offering greater stability during times of change or when working with a past trauma.

WORD TO THE WISE Due to its relationship with the menstrual cycle, do not work with motherwort if you are pregnant.

SUGGESTED PREPARATIONS tincture, body oil

FAVORITE PLANT PAIRINGS skullcap, passionflower, rose, hawthorn, kava

Be Cool Iced Tea

A refreshing and calming blend, drink this whenever it's hot outside and you need a reminder to stay calm, cool, and collected.

MAKES 4 CUPS

1 tablespoon hibiscus
1 tablespoon rose petals
1 tablespoon hawthorn leaf and/or berry
2 teaspoons peppermint
1 teaspoon motherwort

NOTE: All herbs should be cut and sifted.

To make this blend, add all ingredients to a small jar, put the lid on, and shake thoroughly to combine. Label the jar with the blend title, ingredients, and the date you made it. Store the blend out of direct sunlight and it will keep for 8–12 months.

When ready to drink Be Cool Iced Tea, use 1 heaping tablespoon of the blend for every 8 ounces of water. For a single serving, add 1 tablespoon to a reusable tea strainer. Alternatively, you can add the blend to a glass jar or French press and brew up to 32 ounces. Bring water to a boil and pour it over the blend and allow to steep until cool. Strain and pour over ice.

Wood Betony (*Stachys officinalis*)

PARTS USED leaf

ENERGETICS warming, drying

A plant long revered in Europe for its magical and medicinal uses, wood betony has an immediate calming and centering affect, encouraging us to drop into our bodies by stimulating the solar plexus, a complex network of nerves located in the pit of the stomach. Most of us experience a certain level of out-of-bodyness just keeping up with the demands of modern life. If you can't stop thinking and tend to get stuck overanalyzing, if you rarely feel grounded and tend to suffer from mental exhaustion, wood betony is for you. It's a great herbal ally if you tend to rely heavily on your intellect and often feel detached from your body, encouraging you to get in touch with and trust your gut instincts and intuition.

Sometimes embodiment can be difficult; we live in our heads because it feels safer there. Wood betony is ideal for those of us who do not feel entirely safe or accepted in our bodies. There can be many reasons for this, including past trauma that is still held in the body, or not feeling accepted by your loved ones, or oppression due to your size, gender expression, sexuality, race, etc. Wood betony can be helpful for those still processing the lingering effects of trauma or building a practice where they feel safe and protected in their bodies.

WORD TO THE WISE Since so much of your mental health and mood is linked to the health of your digestive system, and more specifically your enteric nervous system or "second brain," working with plants that have an affinity for the nervous and digestive systems is great. Wood betony is an aromatic and bitter mint family herb, assisting our bodies in switching out of a stressed-out, fight-flight-freeze response and into a rest-and-digest response. In addition, regular use of wood betony improves overall digestion while restoring tone to the digestive tissues that can become damaged due to poor diet or food intolerances.

SUGGESTED PREPARATIONS hot infusion, tincture, oxymel

FAVORITE PLANT PAIRINGS St. John's wort, chamomile, rose, damiana, skullcap

Grounded Infusion

If you are feeling spacey, anxious, or detached, brew a cup of this grounding, nourishing infusion. An exceptional blend if you want to relax into intimacy with a partner or drop into your body after a whirlwind week filled with mental exhaustion.

MAKES 4 CUPS

> 2 tablespoons wood betony
> 2 tablespoons nettle
> 1 tablespoon damiana
> 2 teaspoons holy basil/tulsi
> 2 teaspoons hawthorn berry and/or leaf

NOTE: All herbs should be cut and sifted.

To make the blend, add all ingredients to a small jar, put the lid on, and shake thoroughly to combine. Label the jar with the blend title, ingredients, and the date you made it. Store the blend out of direct sunlight and it will keep for 8–12 months.

When ready to drink Grounded Infusion, use 1 heaping tablespoon of the blend for every 8 ounces of water. For a single serving, add 1 tablespoon to a reusable tea strainer. Alternatively, you can add the blend to a glass jar or French press and brew up to 32 ounces. Bring water to a boil and pour it over the blend and allow to steep for a minimum of 15 minutes. Drink hot or refrigerate and enjoy chilled.

Sweet Acceptance Tincture

Sometimes life throws us blows that are hard to accept. These herbs support us as we process the stress and anxiety of big life events. When self-compassion, tenderness, and calm are needed the most, carry this tincture with you.

MAKES 2-OUNCE (60 ML) BOTTLE

20 milliliters wood betony alcohol extract
20 milliliters hawthorn alcohol extract
10 milliliters motherwort alcohol extract
10 milliliters holy basil/tulsi alcohol extract

See page 235 for instructions on making a tincture.

Take 1–2 dropperfuls twice daily for an extended period—minimum 4–6 weeks—to help with overall stress, anxiety, agitation, grief, or depression. In a pinch, for more acute situations, use the pulse-dosing method and take 1–3 dropperfuls whenever anxiety, rage, bitterness, grief, or worry become overwhelming. The tincture can be added to a few inches of drinking water, added to a smoothie or juice, or put directly in the mouth.

Journal Prompts for Stress and Anxiety

→ How are stress and anxiety showing up in your life right now?

→ List the ways you already show up for yourself in moments of heighted stress and anxiety.

→ Are the expectations you have for yourself realistic?

→ Where in your body does stress and anxiety show up? Chest? Neck and shoulders? Digestion? A chronic complaint flare-up?

→ How are you paying attention to the needs of your body? What are they and how can you better listen moving forward?

→ Which herbs and practices can help you to befriend your body?

→ How often do you ask for support?

→ What daily, weekly, and monthly practices are you committed to in order to lower your stress and anxiety?

→ Explore some ways you can create healthy boundaries with social media and technology in general.

→ Brew and drink a quart of Stress Less Infusion (page 106) daily for a full week. How did you feel day to day? What shifted? Did you interact with stressors differently?

→ How can you slow down and declutter your days?

→ List some societal, family, or work norms that might be in direct conflict with your ability to de-stress. What are some healthy ways you can navigate and advocate for your needs within these environments?

→ What foods best support your ability to combat stress and anxiety?

→ Do you need to be productive to feel like you are worthy of love and self-care?

→ What are some boundaries you enact to ensure well-being?

→ What plant allies and practices are you looking forward to incorporating into your self-care?

Relaxation and Sleep

6

IT HAS BECOME TRULY RADICAL to commit yourself to relaxation, rest, and a good night's sleep and know that you are not a bad person for not being able—or not wanting—to keep up with everyone else. Without relaxation and sleep, our health begins to falter, and we have the potential to become more forgetful, stressed, irritable, and moody. When we give ourselves downtime to unwind and get a deep, restful night's sleep, we allow our body time to heal.

If we rest our weary minds and dismantle the notion that productivity is synonymous with self-worth, we would find that the remedies we seek are more often basic lifestyle changes and permission to do less. Herbs are here to help us surrender into the rest we so desperately need, which we tend to forgo due to outside pressures or feeling guilty about taking a break. Once we can surrender to our body's needs, we can begin to say yes to healing our body, mind, and spirit.

Rest and Relaxation

Rest and relaxation are two essential keys to health, but they are often overlooked as we search for a cure-all or quick fix that allows us to continue our unbalanced, busy lifestyle. In fact, many common complaints and diseases stem from an over-stressed nervous system stuck in perpetual fight-flight-freeze mode instead of rest-digest-repair mode.

Instead of reading another article about "life hacks to get more done," perhaps we, individually and as a society, need to consider why we're constantly running around trying to do so much. Is it truly bringing us fulfillment, or are we stuck on a hamster wheel of our own making? Remember, you need leisure time to do all the things you want to do. Rest and relaxation are key to showing up in a way that honors everything you're trying to accomplish in life.

LIFESTYLE

Getting more rest and relaxation doesn't mean being glued to an easy chair, lying around all day in front of the TV. Instead, focus on how you can incorporate more regenerative practices into your life. Whether that's going on an evening walk, people-watching on a bench in the park, reading a good book, riding your bike, spending the day in bed with a lover, taking an afternoon nap, wandering around an art museum, seeing live music, camping, or being creative in your room or among friends, rest and relaxation is entirely based on what makes *you* feel rejuvenated.

Whatever your relaxing activity may be, one crucial piece that should be the undercurrent of achieving more rest and relaxation is slowing down more often. Slowing down allows you to notice the world around you and notice how your body feels day to day. Herbal allies, flower essences, and some lifestyle tweaks will support you tremendously in this pursuit, but you'll also need to pause and consider what's motivating your need to consistently be distracted and on the go. Remember, you're in charge of your life; you're in charge of setting your schedule and asserting your boundaries. So be sure to prioritize some TLC. Try making a list of practices and actions that you can do daily, weekly, and monthly to support you in feeling more rested and rejuvenated.

PRACTICE: IN RELATIONSHIP WITH NATURE

Close your eyes and think back to the last time you were immersed in nature. Can you feel the sun on your skin? Hear the branches of trees swaying in the breeze? Maybe there are birds chirping or the sound of moving water nearby. Do you notice that by mentally journeying back to this moment your breath slows and deepens, the tension in your shoulders melts, and your mind calms?

Most of us are lucky enough to tap into a not-so-distant memory of how deeply rejuvenating it is to get out of the hustle and bustle and be in nature. You might think you have to find some expansive wilderness and own all the right gear, but that's not necessarily so. You can find a moment of peace and calm just watching the clouds float by on your lunch break, properly identifying a plant in your yard, pausing to smell a flower, or sitting under a tree in a park. These experiences connect us with the world through our senses and remind us that the key to relaxation can begin with the simple act of interacting with nature. Here are some other things you can do to connect with nature:

→ Put a pause on screen time and go on a fifteen-minute walk in your neighborhood or local park a few nights a week and see how your mental health shifts. Invite a friend and bring a thermos of tea to share.

→ Bring plants into your home. Invest in houseplants or a small window garden with your favorite medicinal and culinary herbs like mint, oregano, rosemary, or thyme. Or buy fresh flowers to keep at your bedside.

→ Ride a bike for pleasure or your work commute. Getting out of the confines of your car is a great way to engage with the world around you in a more intimate way—not to mention it's great for the environment and your mental and physical health.

→ Nature as works of art: Hang a piece of art in your home depicting beautiful views of trees, flowers, desert landscapes, mountains, or water. Believe it or not, this simple act can impact your well-being.

PRACTICE: THE POWER OF DAILY RITUALS

Daily rituals are an excellent way to infuse your day with a little intention and care. A ritual and a habit aren't too different from each other, though to turn a habit—that is, a task you do unconsciously and without much thought—into a ritual, you need to put a little extra effort and mindfulness into the act.

A ritual carves out space for a little bit of meaning-making and magic in your day. It gets you to slow down and bring awareness to whatever you're doing, which in itself is a powerful act of self-care. Remember, when you slow down, you give your nervous system and your entire body time to integrate all that life is throwing at you, and you'll be able to focus even better on what's important.

> *A ritual carves out space for a little bit of meaning-making and magic in your day. It gets you to slow down and bring awareness to whatever you're doing, which in itself is a powerful act of self-care.*

A ritual could be as simple as lighting a candle to shift the mood of your space as you enjoy your morning coffee and write in your journal, or doing a meditation or tarot card reading for yourself before bed. Try saying affirmations out loud or silently as you take your morning tinctures: "I'm a badass" or "Today is going to be a good day." These little moments can set the tone for how your entire day goes. By taking time to pause and fully experience the things you do throughout the day, you usher in a level of presence and intention that makes the mundane feel special and sacred.

PRACTICE: THE JOY OF MISSING OUT

Perhaps you've heard the acronym FOMO—fear of missing out—a concept built on social anxieties that emphasize that we're missing out on some super-fun experience, inside joke, article, or piece of information that will make us forever regret not being glued to the phone or saying yes to every social engagement. With the advent of social media, even more of us are plagued with the worry that we aren't cool enough or generally doing enough. It's exhausting, isn't it?

This kind of comparison-based thinking can crush our attempts to have a quiet night in and prioritize relaxation and our new favorite self-care practices. This is where the joy of missing out comes in. Or, as I like to call it, the joy of doing exactly what you want to do and not worrying about what everyone else is doing. As long as you're content and enjoying yourself, you're not really missing out on anything, right? Right! This takes practice. It requires taking a step back from social media. It takes firm boundaries and a dedication to self-preservation. It takes wanting to get in touch with yourself and asking, *What do I actually want to be doing? What do I need in this moment?* And it takes having the confidence, self-love, and courage to put that in motion.

Let's face it, the fear of missing out is real and very human. We all want to be included. From an evolutionary standpoint, being cast out of the community carried the possibility of being a death sentence, as our ancestors very much depended on one another for basic survival. The need to belong is deeply embedded in us, yet modern life as dictated by social calendars and to-do lists is a far cry from the lives of our not-so-distant ancestors.

You have to confront a certain level of fear in order to advocate for your needs. The people who love you will get it.

HERBS AND FLOWER ESSENCES

Many of the herbs mentioned in chapters 4 and 5 can be of great use in reestablishing your relationship with rest and relaxation. Restorative tonic herbs like ashwagandha, gotu kola, holy basil/tulsi, milky oat, nettle, oatstraw, and reishi nourish the body, while blue vervain, California poppy, chamomile, kava, lavender, lemon balm, passionflower, skullcap, rose, and wood betony offer more calming effects for those who have trouble soothing the mind, letting go of tension, and relaxing the body.

If you want to work with flower essences for rest and relaxation, start with bougainvillea or jumping cholla cactus. Bougainvillea flower essence relaxes the body and deepens our breathing, encouraging feelings of ease and calm. Jumping cholla cactus flower essence aids us in fostering inner calm. It can be used to help with frenzied running around, to help us respond rather than react. When taking action is informed by obsessive worry or feelings of urgency, jumping cholla steadies and calms, reminding us there's no need to rush.

Skullcap (*Scutellaria lateriflora*)

PARTS USED leaf

ENERGETICS cooling

A versatile and effective herb, skullcap is a nervous-system restorative that subtly shifts how you experience stress so you feel capable of rolling with life's punches. Skullcap can be enjoyed over a long period of time without any ill effects, so you can build a daily practice with it. Unlike some herbs, skullcap will not cause any drowsiness and can be used throughout the day. It benefits those dealing with anxiety, nervousness, worry, chronic fatigue, and insomnia. People who are sensitive to stimulation like light, sounds, and touch, or who are easily overwhelmed by crowds will benefit from skullcap. Carry a tincture along with you to take as needed and savor a cup of tea after any stressful outing to further relax.

In the wake of a great shock, skullcap is an indispensable herbal ally. Whether an unexpected personal upset or a collective tragedy has shaken up your life, skullcap will reinforce your foundation. It is also a remedy for general body pains, injuries, and cramps and will soothe both the physical pain and mental irritation of your circumstance. Skullcap can also amplify the efficacy of other herbs like kava, passionflower, and valerian for severe or chronic pain.

WORD TO THE WISE Fresh plant preparations tend to be more restorative to the nervous system, while dry plant preparations are more sedating, assisting in issues like sleeplessness or anxiety.

SUGGESTED PREPARATIONS hot infusion, tincture

FAVORITE PLANT PAIRINGS oatstraw, valerian, passionflower, kava, blue vervain

Sustained Calm Infusion

Create a daily tea ritual with this beloved infusion. An uplifting, nervous system–fortifying, sweet blend full of nourishing and heartfelt support. Long-term use will encourage mental and emotional resilience, support digestive health, and regulate mood.

MAKES 4 CUPS

1 tablespoon passionflower

1 tablespoon lemon balm

1 tablespoon skullcap

2 teaspoons rose petals

2 teaspoons catnip

NOTE: All herbs should be cut and sifted.

To make the blend, add all ingredients to a small jar, put the lid on, and shake thoroughly to combine. Label the jar with the blend title, ingredients, and the date you made it. Store the blend out of direct sunlight and it will keep for 8–12 months.

When ready to drink Sustained Calm Infusion, use 1 heaping tablespoon of the blend for every 8 ounces of water. For a single serving, add 1 tablespoon to a reusable tea strainer. Alternatively, you can add the blend to a glass jar or French press and brew up to 32 ounces. Bring water to a boil and pour it over the blend and allow it to steep for a minimum of 15 minutes. Drink hot or refrigerate and enjoy chilled.

Joy of Missing Out Tincture

This tincture will help quiet the voice of comparison that says you must be constantly doing, going, and keeping up. To help replenish your reserves, fortify your sense of self, support your boundaries and ability to advocate and prioritize your needs—this is a no-is-a-full-sentence kind of tincture.

MAKES 2-OUNCE (60 ML) BOTTLE

25 milliliters holy basil/tulsi alcohol extract
10 milliliters skullcap alcohol extract
10 milliliters hawthorn alcohol extract
5 milliliters blue vervain alcohol extract
5 milliliters reishi alcohol extract
5 drops oak flower essence
5 drops yarrow flower essence

See page 235 for instructions on making a tincture.

Take 1–2 dropperfuls twice daily for an extended period—minimum 4–6 weeks—to help with overall feelings of comparison, self-worth, a lack of boundaries, or anxiety. In a pinch, for more acute situations, take 2–4 dropperfuls whenever FOMO is at its worst. This tincture can be added to a few inches of drinking water, added to a smoothie or juice, or put directly in the mouth.

Chamomile (*Matricaria recutita*)

PARTS USED flower

ENERGETICS cooling

From ancient Egypt to the Middle Ages in Europe, this delicate flower has made its mark throughout the centuries and in cultures across the world. In Mexico its Spanish name is *manzanilla*, meaning "little apple," which refers to the apple-like scent of the flowers. Before you even ingest chamomile you can breathe in its sweet fragrance and experience a deep sense of calm and tranquility. The mild bitterness of a chamomile infusion improves digestion while its aromatics comfort stomach complaints. Chamomile reduces inflammation internally and externally, bringing effective, all-around treatment for a wide variety of ailments.

Chamomile reminds us to be tender and compassionate with ourselves in times of struggle and to release what no longer serves our greater good. It has a special ability to relax nerves and muscles throughout the body so we can better unwind. A simple tea can offer support in moments of stress, anxiety, nervous tension, insomnia, and overwhelm, especially when symptoms manifest as digestive issues like gas, ulcers, or indigestion. A foot soak or warm bath of chamomile and Epsom salts will ease muscle and joint pain and can be a supportive weekly ritual for those with chronic pain, as with arthritis or fibromyalgia. In addition, count on chamomile to relieve moodiness, tension, and cramps due to PMS. Enjoy it alone or combine with lemon balm and rose when you or a loved one is in a grumpy, agitated mood.

WORD TO THE WISE For some people with sensitivities to ragweed, chamomile can cause similar allergic reactions. Though this is rare, pay attention to any signs or symptoms when first interacting with this plant.

SUGGESTED PREPARATIONS hot infusion or tea, tincture, herbal bath, oxymel

FAVORITE PLANT PAIRINGS lemon balm, fennel, calendula, marshmallow root

Chamomile and Mugwort Dream Oil

Whenever you feel tense and full of worry, reach for this oil blend to massage into the soles of your feet, neck, shoulders, and temples before drifting off to dreamland.

MAKES 8-OUNCE JAR

3 tablespoons mugwort
3 tablespoons chamomile
1 cup carrier oil(s) of choice

NOTE: All herbs should be cut and sifted.

See page 237 for instructions on making herbal oil.

To use, massage a quarter-sized amount into hands and massage into clean, dry skin, prioritizing areas that are sore or typically hold stress and tension like the feet, neck, and shoulders. You may wish to anoint your temples as well. This oil can be used to release tension and encourage restful sleep and dreaming.

NOTE: Some of my favorite carrier oils are organic, cold-pressed, unrefined sesame, olive, almond, argan, and apricot kernel. Pick one or combine several.

Joyful Surrender Infusion

Uplifting, relaxing, aromatic, and floral, this blend will aid you in cultivating self-compassion, softening you into relaxation while reminding you to stop and smell the roses.

MAKES 4 CUPS

2 tablespoons chamomile

2 tablespoons lemon balm

2 teaspoons passionflower

2 teaspoons hawthorn berry and/or leaf

2 teaspoons rose petals

NOTE: All herbs should be cut and sifted.

To make the blend, add all ingredients to a small jar, put the lid on, and shake thoroughly to combine. Label the jar with the blend title, ingredients, and the date you made it. Store the blend out of direct sunlight and it will keep for 8–12 months.

When ready to drink Joyful Surrender Infusion, use 1 heaping tablespoon of the blend for every 8 ounces of water. For a single serving, add 1 tablespoon to a reusable tea strainer. Alternatively, you can add the blend to a glass jar or French press and brew up to 32 ounces. Bring water to a boil and pour it over the blend and allow to steep for a minimum of 15 minutes. Drink hot or refrigerate and enjoy chilled.

Sleeplessness and Insomnia

From the occasional restless night to a more longstanding disruption in your sleep patterns, sleep issues can be a real problem for many. Insomnia can be understood as insufficient, disturbed, unrestorative sleep and can be classified in various ways, from being caused by physical or psychological complaints, to side effects from a medication, to poor diet and lifestyle habits. There are various forms of sleeplessness. For instance, you might be the type who falls asleep as soon as your head hits the pillow, but you find yourself up and alert hours later feeling agitated. Others can't fall asleep if their life depended on it. Luckily, in either situation, herbs, as well as a few dietary and lifestyle changes, can help.

There isn't a one-size-fits-all approach for how much sleep a person needs. What matters most is that you're able to rise in the morning rested and ready to take on the day. For some, that means a solid eight or nine hours, while others feel perfectly fine with five or six. This can sometimes vary as the seasons change. During the winter months it isn't uncommon to find yourself craving more sleep and downtime, as the sun sets earlier and our natural inclination is to hibernate and sleep longer. Always trust what feels best for you.

LIFESTYLE

First and foremost, reduce stress, as stress often plays a big part in sleep disturbances. Identify the stressors in your life and establish practices or seek out professional guidance that can support you in navigating or removing them. Daily exercise and community engagement will help dispel physical and mental energy, while yoga, breathwork, meditation, an evening walk, or a foot soak or bath will help calm and rejuvenate a wired nervous system. Notice any unhealthy dietary habits, like eating large, heavy meals before bedtime or drinking alcohol late into the evening, as both stimulate the liver and digestion in general, causing sleep disturbances. Set boundaries around your sleep schedule and unplug before bedtime, keeping screens like cell phones, computers, tablets, and TVs out of the bedroom. At the very least, do not use them an hour before bedtime as the light from electronic devices can throw the body off its natural sleep rhythms. Finally, create a before-bed sleep ritual with herbs like ashwagandha.

PRACTICE: SNACKS FOR SLEEP

For those who feel too stressed and wired to settle into sleep, a small, protein-packed snack—say, a hardboiled egg with sea salt, a cup of Ashwagandha Golden Milk (page 85), or some nuts—can help absorb excess stress hormones in the blood so you can relax and more easily drift off to sleep. To this day, my mom favors a bowl of cereal when plagued with restlessness. Whole milk and grains always settle her for a good night's sleep.

PRACTICE: CREATING A BEDTIME RITUAL WITH HERBS

If insomnia or trouble getting to sleep is a chronic issue, create a sleep ritual in the hour or two before going to bed.

Limit screen time and don't engage in anything that will overly excite or stress your system. An hour or so before bedtime, take 1–2 dropperfuls of Restful Slumber Tincture (page 138) or a sleep tincture of your choice while brewing a cup of grounding, relaxing tea like Skullcap Bedtime Infusion (page 127) or Sweet Heart Infusion (page 151). Quietly sip the tea and take another 1–2 dropperfuls of sleep tincture. About 10–15 minutes before your desired bedtime, check in with how you're feeling. If you still feel restless, wired, or wide awake, up the tincture dosage to 2–3 dropperfuls. Once again, depending on how you feel, as you get into bed, take 1–3 more dropperfuls (if you already feel sleepy, there's no need to continue taking the tincture). This is called *pulse dosing*, and is often recommended by herbalists for acute situations like insomnia and anxiety. Read more about pulse dosing with acute remedies in chapter 5 (page 111).

For those who find it easy to fall asleep but tend to wake up in the early hours of the morning, work with a combination of herbs like ashwagandha, holy basil/tulsi, and passionflower for 4–6 weeks.

HERBS AND FLOWER ESSENCES

Depending on the severity of your sleep issues, you may decide to work with several formulas or seek support from a trained clinical herbalist who can assist you in pinpointing the root cause.

Sleep disturbances can be related to an imbalance in one's internal rhythms, known as *circadian rhythms*, which are affected by the nervous and endocrine systems. Work with a tonic formula including adaptogens (ashwagandha, holy basil/tulsi, licorice), nutritives (oat, nettle), and gently calming, nervous system–strengthening herbs (chamomile, damiana, lavender, lemon balm, linden, rose, skullcap).

These herbs can be taken as an infusion or tincture 2–3 times daily. A secondary, acute formula like Lights-Out Sleep Tincture (page 136) can be taken strictly before bedtime, for example, as part of a bedtime ritual (page 133). Stronger sedative and relaxing herbs include, but are not limited to, California poppy, hops, kava, passionflower, and valerian.

If you want to work with flower essences for sleeplessness and insomnia, try white chestnut and valerian to start. White chestnut flower essence can be used for mental chatter, those thoughts and worries that keep you up at night. It also pairs nicely with passionflower tincture. Valerian flower essence is excellent for those agitated, irritable states that leave you feeling unfocused and frustrated. It helps to transform anger and rage into fertile emotions instead of allowing them to fester and cause sleep issues.

Dosing for Sleep Disturbances

Once you find an herb or blend of herbs to help with sleep, consider how best to take the herbs so you can get the most out of them. Depending on the severity of your insomnia or sleeplessness, a soothing cup of herbal tea might do the trick, or you may need to repeatedly take a large dose of a tincture leading up to bedtime, known as pulse dosing.

As always, make sure you address any underlying causes, such as stress, unresolved emotional disturbances, hormone imbalance, late-night drinking, and so forth. Herbs will only do so much if the root cause of the imbalance is not dealt with.

Valerian (*Valeriana officinalis*)

PARTS USED root

ENERGETICS warming

Valerian is one of the best-known and reliable herbs for relaxing the nervous system. It is also a great herbal reminder of the importance of matching your personal constitution to plant energetics. You might have already noticed that valerian is one of the few warming nervines. While valerian is one of the best herbal sleep remedies and acts as a potent sedative for most people, some encounter the opposite effect and end up feeling a bit stimulated, making sleep more difficult to come by. If you're someone who loves to pile on the blankets and tends to always be a little chilled, with cold hands and feet, valerian is probably your sleep remedy of choice. If you generally kick off all the blankets and run warm at night, there is a higher chance that valerian will cause the opposite desired effect. The best thing to do when starting to work with valerian is to take a small dose (a few drops, up to 1 dropperful) during the day or a few hours before bedtime. If you notice any agitation or stimulating effects, this sleep remedy may not be suited for you.

Oftentimes you will find valerian in formulas with cooling herbs like hops, passionflower, or skullcap, as these herbs balance valerian's energetics. In fact, pairing hops and valerian is a beloved sleep remedy for many herbalists. Together, these two herbs make an even more formidable medicine for deep sleep.

WORD TO THE WISE Some people notice a slight groggy feeling the morning after taking valerian. You may consider experimenting with a tincture on its own to determine how it will best support your sleep before adding valerian to a sleep blend.

SUGGESTED PREPARATIONS tincture, capsule, or flower essence

FAVORITE PLANT PAIRINGS hops, passionflower, skullcap

Lights-Out Sleep Tincture

This formula is ideal if you're needing a little extra something to help you get to sleep, and it should be taken in the hours leading up to bedtime. Valerian, hops, and passionflower combine to make a wonderfully sedating formula that will induce sleep when you need it most.

MAKES 2-OUNCE (60 ML) BOTTLE

20 milliliters valerian alcohol extract
20 milliliters hops alcohol extract
20 milliliters passionflower alcohol extract

See page 235 for instructions on making a tincture.

In a pinch, for more acute situations, use the pulse-dosing method mentioned on page 26 and take 2–4 dropperfuls whenever you're having trouble sleeping. The tincture can be added to a few inches of drinking water, added to a smoothie or juice, or put directly in the mouth.

Hops for Sleep

Hops is a dependable, sedating, pain-relieving sleep herb. It can be especially helpful for folks who tend to drink alcohol—specifically beer—before bedtime in an attempt to self-medicate and get to sleep. Since they already have a relationship with hops, which is used to make beer, this herb can be a supportive transition out of an unhealthy dependency on alcohol.

Passionflower (*Passiflora incarnata*)

PARTS USED flower, leaf

ENERGETICS cooling

Passionflower, affectionately known as *maypop* in the southern states where it grows, is an eye-catching flowering vine with a calming effect on the central nervous system. Passionflower is commonly used for restlessness; mental, physical, and emotional agitation; and an inability to sink into relaxation due to chronic stress or general overexertion. For those fiery, driven types who are prone to burnout and eschew taking any time off, passionflower is the chill pill they so desperately need. In addition, this cooling remedy can benefit anyone with a tendency to get irritable, moody, or hotheaded when they are stressed.

Passionflower is excellent alone or in combination with other herbs for hypertension, anxiety, nerve pain, or insomnia. Use passionflower after a fun night out, when you're back at home and need to get some sleep but feel too worked up. When you can't get to sleep because you're stuck analyzing conversations from the past week, anticipating everything that must get done the next day, or simply because you're worrying about not being able to sleep, call on passionflower. Passionflower does not force sleep; rather, it gently lulls us to sleep without any sedative hangover the next day.

WORD TO THE WISE Passionflower is an herbal synergist, meaning that when combined with other herbs for sleep, anxiety, or stress, it enhances the potency of the other herbs, making the blend better than a single herb.

SUGGESTED PREPARATIONS tincture, tea, herbal bath

FAVORITE PLANT PAIRINGS skullcap, valerian, hops, chamomile

Restful Slumber Tincture

A balancing, system-replenishing formula, this can be taken throughout the day as a tonic or in higher doses before bedtime to encourage restful sleep and calm. This formula will also help shift any longstanding, chronic stress or health issues that might be causing sleep disturbances.

MAKES 2-OUNCE (60 ML) BOTTLE

20 milliliters passionflower alcohol extract
20 milliliters ashwagandha alcohol extract
15 milliliters milky oat alcohol extract
5 milliliters lavender alcohol extract

See page 235 for instructions on making a tincture.

Take 1–2 dropperfuls twice daily for an extended period—minimum 4–6 weeks—to help with overall energy levels, restlessness, fatigue, insomnia, mental chatter, or stress. In a pinch, for more acute situations, use the pulse-dosing method and take 2–4 dropperfuls whenever you need support falling asleep and staying asleep.

Skullcap Bedtime Infusion

Let the stress of the day melt away by enjoying a cup of this infusion in the hour or so before bed as part of a sleep ritual. This blend helps you to sink into relaxation, release tension, and promote calm.

MAKES 4 CUPS

2 tablespoons skullcap

1 tablespoon passionflower

1 tablespoon oatstraw

2 teaspoons mint (any variety)

1 teaspoon lavender

NOTE: All herbs should be cut and sifted.

To make the blend, add all ingredients to a small jar, put the lid on, and shake thoroughly to combine. Label the jar with the blend title, ingredients, and the date you made it. Store the blend out of direct sunlight and it will keep for 8–12 months.

When ready to drink Skullcap Bedtime Infusion, use 1 heaping tablespoon of the blend for every 8 ounces of water. For a single serving, add 1 tablespoon to a reusable tea strainer. Alternatively, you can add the blend to a glass jar or French press and brew up to 32 ounces. Bring water to a boil and pour it over the blend and allow to steep for a minimum of 15 minutes. Drink hot or refrigerate and enjoy chilled.

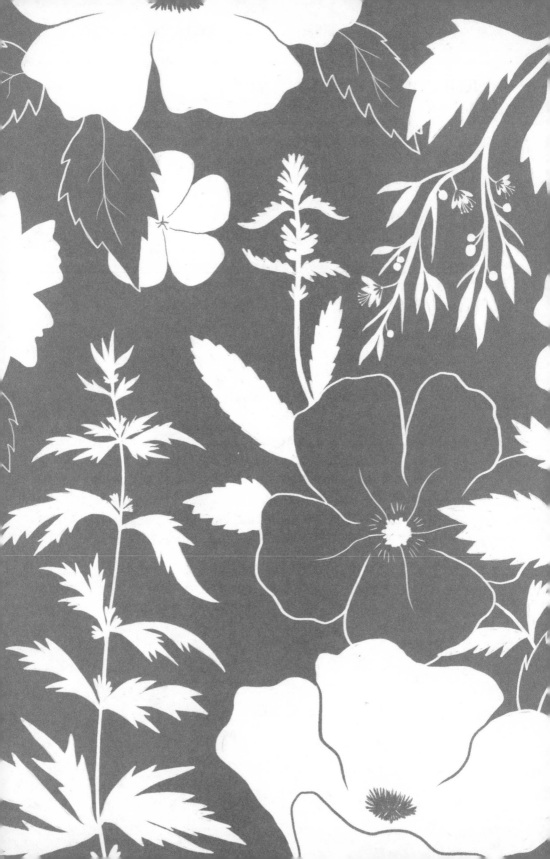

Emotional Well-Being

7

I DON'T KNOW ABOUT YOU, but when I'm having a tough time I tend to feel alone and can get pretty hard on myself. It's easy to want to hide away, but that only intensifies the feelings of isolation and melancholy. There are also the things that get us down that seem so much bigger than us, like sexism, homophobia, transphobia, racism, genocide, war, pollution, and global warming. Even if we wake up every day with an understanding that on an individual level we are healthy, happy, and grateful, we are interconnected with the greater natural and cultural world that is undergoing immense pressures. As sensitive beings, it's no wonder we feel a level of sadness due to the state of the world.

Although we can't change these things on our own or overnight, the good news is that you don't have to do it alone, and even when you live alone you can still be supported by plants and the natural world. Medicinal herbs can come to your aid. They can be your support system; you can sit with them, process your feelings with them, and move through difficult emotions with their help. Herbs, along with a healthy diet, can strengthen your personal foundation, reminding you that radical change starts from within, with compassionate acts of self-care that ripple out.

When we welcome plants into our lives, we feel connected to the world around us in an intimate, personal way. Connecting with nature—the phases of the moon, the first buds of spring, the buzzing of bees in late summer—brings our world into greater balance and wards off loneliness. It's through your relationships with medicinal herbs—growing them, sitting with them, making medicines with them, and ingesting them—that you, and perhaps the world, can begin to heal.

Plants and Pills

The reality is, most people nowadays are on some sort of medication, so we're not suggesting you should forsake your meds and only work with plants. In fact, there's nothing wrong with taking pharmaceuticals and finding support from conventional medicine. We should try to break down any judgment we may have about people who take pharmaceuticals in an effort to sustain optimal physical and mental health. Attaching these kinds of stigmas further isolates people at a time when we as friends, family members, lovers, and community members should come together and praise them for the courage they're taking to seek help.

That said, the power of Big Pharma is wildly out of control, their lobbying groups are mainly concerned with shareholders' profits over genuine care. This has led to certain health-care providers overprescribing pharmaceutical drugs and the drug companies themselves charging an arm and a leg for life-sustaining medications that people need, often exploiting poor or marginalized communities in the process. This must become a national conversation as we fight for access to health care as a basic human right. In the meantime, there is no reason to harshly judge ourselves or others if conventional treatments and medications are needed.

In the end, health isn't about forsaking plants for pills or vice versa; it's about building a relationship with both that allows you to move through life confidently. Both have their place in health care and can be indispensable tools when used appropriately and with respect.

Difficult Emotions

We've all been there. Heartbreak, grief, anger, hurt feelings, and other difficult emotions are all part of life. Nowadays we live in an uncertain world, so it's no surprise that as we move through life we will confront personal and collective struggles and emotional turmoil. Fortunately, there are plenty of ways you can support yourself.

→ Eat nutritious food.

→ Surround yourself with a supportive community.

→ Prioritize pleasure and play.

→ Channel your emotions through political action, exercise, and creative expression.

→ Take time for self-inquiry and contemplation.

→ Invest in herbs that relieve stress and fortify your tender heart.

→ Incorporate practices that help you sit with, process, and move through difficult emotions.

Difficult emotions are hard to talk about openly. There's a level of taboo and stigma that comes with speaking openly about feelings of depression, loss, grief, shame, anger, and bitterness, and very often people feel very isolated with these feelings. However, that's when you most need a support system. When we don't deal with difficult emotions in a healthy way, they have the potential to choke joy and stifle vitality; they fester and cause harm not only to ourselves but also to those we love.

We've largely been taught that what we feel can't be trusted, that speaking from a place of feeling makes us irrational, weak, or overly sensitive. When we pretend that we're fine when we're not, we numb ourselves to our own truth. But shutting down in this way prevents us from becoming whole and healthy. Moreover, when we don't deal with emotions in a healthy way, it not only impacts us personally but the greater world as well. In fact, traumatic life events and hardships and the emotions they bring up have the ability to literally change one's DNA, and in this way painful emotions are passed down through the generations. Shame is a good example. Much like stress and all the other difficult emotions, it can cause inflammation and negatively affect one's physical and mental well-being.

So it's vitally important that we show up to address our difficult emotions with compassion and curiosity so they do not control us and thereby negatively impact others and future generations.

When we invest in our emotional well-being, when we take time to understand our inner landscape so that we can better communicate our needs, we claim our ability to be whole. By nurturing our whole selves—emotional, mental, physical, and spiritual—we open up a new channel of thought and feeling that empowers us and allows us to stay firmly rooted in our complexity as human beings.

LIFESTYLE

When you're experiencing a difficult emotion, one of the best things you can do is to process and move through the emotion, letting go of it so that it doesn't hold you prisoner. Of course, not every emotion caused by trauma, loss, heartbreak, or setback will be easy to move on from. It takes curiosity, humor, personal inquiry, and sometimes professional support to understand and work through these experiences. It's not so much about moving on but finding healthy ways to accept what you're feeling and sitting with the difficult emotions. Sometimes that process can take years or even a lifetime.

Contemplative and movement practices are excellent tools for processing emotions. Some of these include:

→ Breathwork (page 109)

→ Pulling tarot or oracle cards

→ Prayer (or any intention-setting or gratitude-focused practice)

→ Time spent in nature (page 123)

→ Mindfulness meditation

→ Free writing (page 145)

→ Cooking

→ Restorative yoga (199)

→ Dance

→ Regular exercise

→ Taking a walk

→ Gardening

→ Chanting and singing

→ Doing art

In particular, mindfulness meditation, free writing, and breathwork can do wonders if you tend to react impulsively and hurt people close to you. These practices strengthen the parts of your brain that help you remain calm under pressure and react less to adverse situations, giving you time to consider how your words or actions will affect others and the long-term consequences.

Depending on your circumstances, the enormity of your feelings, and the impact on your day-to-day life and relationships, you may find it necessary to seek support from a mental health professional. I cannot recommend this enough. Practitioners best suited to helping people work through difficult emotions include:

Radical Remedies

- → Trauma-informed massage therapists
- → Craniofacial- or myofascial-release practitioners
- → Trained, trauma-informed herbalists
- → Therapists and counselors
- → EMDR (eye movement desensitization and reprocessing) practitioners
- → Reiki practitioners
- → Breathwork practitioners

PRACTICE: FREE WRITING

Free writing is often recommended as a technique to help writers and artists move through creative blocks. In this same way, it can be a useful tool to help any of us begin to process emotions, identifying themes or conclusions in a nonjudgmental, raw way. This stream-of-consciousness practice can be done by journaling or writing a letter you don't plan to send. Try writing for a certain amount of time without pause, say fifteen minutes, or writing a certain number of pages, say three. The point is to let your mind go and not censor yourself in any way. A reflective, flowing, liberating practice, free writing is incredibly cathartic and illuminating when done as a daily ritual. Light a candle, brew a cup of herbal tea, and just write whatever comes into your mind. Think of how difficult emotions weigh on you, how they infiltrate your interactions with others and affect your vitality and well-being. Giving yourself time every day to write about what you think and feel unburdens you and can offer insight into where or how self-compassion, forgiveness, and healing can arise.

> Light a candle, brew a cup of herbal tea, and
> just write whatever comes into your mind.

You could also try pulling a tarot or oracle card to get you started. What does the imagery bring up for you? Begin to write and stay curious and nonjudgmental about what arises. Don't worry about grammar or spelling, about making sense or writing fully formed thoughts. Just get it out on the paper. If you have a plant ally or formula that you've been working with, you may wish to take that before you start writing to guide or support the practice.

HERBS AND FLOWER ESSENCES

Some of my favorite herbs to work with are those that have an affinity for or effect on the emotional, or energetic, heart. Unlike the physical heart, which is responsible for pumping blood and supplying the body with oxygen and nutrients, the emotional heart resides in a more poetic or metaphorical place. This doesn't lessen its importance in one's well-being in the slightest. We all know the depth of hurt when someone has broken our heart, the grief of losing someone we love, or the sting of getting laid off from work. Even though we know the physical muscle is still working, emotionally the heart is breaking, setting in motion more difficult emotions and stress.

Work with heart healers and openers like rose and hawthorn when you feel raw, vulnerable, hurt, shattered, grief-stricken, angry, or unable to release and forgive. For those who tend to be overly critical of themselves and others, these medicines of the heart can remind you to be gentle and compassionate.

> Unlike the physical heart, which is responsible
> for pumping blood and supplying the body with
> oxygen and nutrients, the emotional heart resides
> in a more poetic or metaphorical place.

If you are excited about a new crush or eager to start dating after a tough breakup, add rose or hawthorn (or both) to your daily self-care, as these plants will encourage you when you are feeling fearful or nervous about opening up to someone or something new. Likewise, if you are working on self-love, these plants can be added to the mix to bestow more kindness and self-acceptance as you move through your day.

If you want to work with flower essences for difficult emotions, try bleeding heart and borage to start. Bleeding heart aids us in healing the heartbreak and grief that comes with a loss of connection, whether due to a breakup or death, encouraging us to see the spiritual lessons. If you find yourself needing to get out of an emotionally abusive or codependent relationship or state of mind, bleeding heart can offer the conviction needed to untangle yourself. Borage lifts you out of the heaviness of emotional, physical, or spiritual upset and offers a newfound optimism and lightness. For long-held sorrow, depression, anger, and grief that weighs you down, borage is heartfelt courage.

Hawthorn (*Crataegus* spp.)

PARTS USED flower, leaf, berry, thorn

ENERGETICS cooling, moistening

The heart is the source of so much of our power and purpose. Hawthorn is a member of the Rosaceae, or rose, family, and like rose it shares an affinity for heart healing. Hawthorn is a heart tonic that strengthens both the physical and emotional heart. Rich in antioxidants, this herb is a cardiac tonic that can nourish and protect the heart and circulatory system and can be used as a preventative or recovery agent if heart disease or heart attack runs in your family.

Hawthorn is a kindhearted ally in moments of grief and heartbreak, holding us in our anguish and soothing our hurt. For those who have a difficult time expressing their emotions, sip hawthorn and rose tea as you share. Hawthorn calms and centers you into your being, quieting an overactive, anxious mind while allowing your heart to take the reins.

Hawthorn is a boundary plant that can be especially helpful for those who feel like their worth is wrapped up in being what others need. You can combine it with yarrow if your work has you immersed in other people's energies. Hawthorn can help you discern what's right for you, trust your heart, and find courage in moments of asking for what you need.

WORD TO THE WISE Dried hawthorn berries, thorns, or a small branch can make a beautiful addition to an altar to set heart-healing intentions, or added to a medicine pouch and worn for heart protection and boundaries.

SUGGESTED PREPARATIONS tea, tincture, syrup, talisman

FAVORITE PLANT PAIRINGS rose, passionflower, skullcap, motherwort, damiana

Heart Renewal Tincture

A calming, heart-nourishing, anxiety-soothing blend. This tincture is an ideal support during the weeks and months following heartbreak and loss, anger and upset.

MAKES 2-OUNCE (60 ML) BOTTLE

30 milliliters hawthorn leaf and/or berry alcohol extract

15 milliliters motherwort alcohol extract

10 milliliters hawthorn rose honey

5–10 drops bleeding heart flower essence

See page 235 for instructions on making a tincture.

Take 1–2 dropperfuls twice daily for an extended period—minimum 2–4 weeks—to help with feelings of shame, heartbreak, anger, resentment, or grief. In a pinch, for more acute situations, take 2–4 dropperfuls whenever you feel overwhelmed. This tincture can be added to a few inches of drinking water, added to a smoothie or juice, or put directly in the mouth.

Hawthorn Rose Honey

A sweet, heart-focused honey that promotes self-kindness and compassion as you move through upheaval, heartache, and loss.
MAKES 8-OUNCE JAR

3 tablespoons hawthorn berry, flower, and/or leaf
2 tablespoons rose petals
1 cup local raw honey

NOTE: All herbs should be cut and sifted.

See page 229 for instructions on making herbal honey.

Enjoy this honey by the spoonful when you need to soften your inner critic, soothe the stress and pain of a breakup, have a difficult conversation with a loved one, or when experiencing bitterness, grief, rage, or self-hatred. Add to tea or enjoy by the spoonful to bring a much-needed smile to your face. This honey is mood-elevating and heart-softening! Honey can be stored in a cool, dark place or in the fridge.

NOTE: Children under one year old should not be given honey.

Rose (*Rosa* spp.)

PARTS USED flower, fruit (known as rose hips)

ENERGETICS cooling, drying

As a heart healer and opener, this lovely, sacred flower reminds us to stay open and aware of all the love in our lives. With its thorns and blossoms, rose carries lessons of boldness, beauty, and boundaries. In one way or another we have all known the difficulty of reclaiming our wholeness and learning to love again in the aftermath of loss. Rose reinforces self-love and personal empowerment, lifting our spirits so we believe in our worth. Rose is a balancing, cooling herb ideal for treating constitutionally hot conditions or those that have a tendency to be hard on themselves. Rose is a nudge toward self-forgiveness as we move through our emotions, especially the more difficult feelings that we're often taught are unacceptable to experience or express, and therefore become repressed or stuck within us.

Rose petals in honey are a cherished delight; add a spoonful to a cup of tea or to satisfy a sweet tooth. Rose honey is also a surprising first-aid ally for stings and burns. Instead of a bandage, place a honeyed rose petal on the wound. Rose-infused vinegar is a remedy for sunburn or inflamed skin. A nightly skin-care ritual is to spray rose water, also known as rose hydrosol, on freshly cleaned skin, allow to air dry, and gently massage a few drops of calendula-infused rose hip oil on the skin. Internally, rose is a soothing remedy for the inflamed tissue of the gut.

WORD TO THE WISE Rose hips, which are the fruit of the plant, are packed with vitamin C, thus boosting the immune system. Rose hip syrup is a delicious way to get an extra immune boost.

SUGGESTED PREPARATIONS honey with petals and/or hips, hydrosol, hot infusion, bath

FAVORITE PLANT PAIRINGS hawthorn, wood betony, elderberry, ginger, lemon balm

Sweet Heart Infusion

A lovely pairing that can't be beat. Relaxing, cooling, heart-soothing, floral, and uplifting goodness. Excellent iced on a sweltering summer day or hot during the dark winter months when melancholy and listlessness increase.

MAKES 4 CUPS

2 tablespoons lemon balm
2 tablespoons rose petals
1 tablespoon hawthorn berry and/or leaf

NOTE: All herbs should be cut and sifted.

To make the blend, add all ingredients to a small jar, put the lid on, and shake thoroughly to combine. Label the jar with the blend title, ingredients, and the date you made it. Store the blend out of direct sunlight and it will keep for 8–12 months.

When ready to drink Sweet Heart Infusion, use 1 heaping tablespoon of the blend for every 8 ounces of water. For a single serving, add 1 tablespoon to a reusable tea strainer. Alternatively, you can add the blend to a glass jar or French press and brew up to 32 ounces. Bring water to a boil and pour it over the blend and allow it to steep for a minimum of 15 minutes. Drink hot or refrigerate and enjoy chilled.

Release Grief Tincture

A supportive blend to comfort you as you move through grief and loss. Gentle and deeply fortifying to body, mind, and spirit.

MAKES 4-OUNCE (120 ML) BOTTLE

> 40 milliliters reishi alcohol extract
> 45 milliliters milky oat alcohol extract
> 20 milliliters rose alcohol extract
> 5 milliliters elecampane alcohol extract
> 5–10 drops borage, bleeding heart, and/ or pink yarrow
> flower essence

See page 235 for instructions on making a tincture.

Take 1–2 dropperfuls twice daily for an extended period—minimum 4–6 weeks—to help process feelings of grief, shock, anger, heartbreak, fatigue, nervousness, or depression. This tincture is nurturing during a spiritual crisis or traumatic event, whether you're presently going through it or reliving and working through the experience in therapy. This tincture can be added to a few inches of drinking water, added to a smoothie or juice, or put directly in the mouth.

Depression

We've all experienced, or love someone who has experienced, depression at some point. Whether it's the occasional case of the blues, a touch of melancholy and listlessness after a personal hardship or in response to current events, that yearly bout of seasonal depression when the daylight dims, or a more longstanding battle with severe depression, we all have our own unique story.

Depression doesn't have one cause, so working with herbs, diet, and lifestyle is an ideal approach to targeting the many internal and external causes that are often involved in depression. Herbs can help you isolate the independent issues and treat each one as they arise. For some, it's a matter of good vitamin D supplementation in the wintertime. For others, it's removing or lessening inflammatory foods like dairy, gluten, or sugar. And for others, deep-seated trauma and an ancestral history of depression might require counseling from a qualified therapist or trained herbalist as well as other forms of community and professional support.

LIFESTYLE

Because depression is such an individual issue, it can be tricky to make recommendations that will work for everyone. Diet, lifestyle changes, and herbal support can be extremely helpful, though it is important to be patient with yourself as it often takes weeks to a few months or even years to experience significant results.

Daily exercise can play a huge role in shifting out of a depressed, depleted, or stagnant state. Start slow with a restorative or yin yoga class (page 199) and evening walks if energy levels are low and lethargy is a problem. Community engagement, monthly bodywork, or regular therapy, as well as self-love practices, plenty of time to relax without judgment, and a good night sleep are also important.

For many, depression is cloaked in shame. It's common to want to isolate when we're not feeling our best. In fact, many people don't ask for support because they don't want to burden their loved ones. But remember—self-care doesn't mean figuring it out all by yourself. It can be helpful to find a trained herbalist or other health-care professional in your area to guide you in identifying the underlying causes of your depression. In talking with a professional, you may begin to notice patterns that you didn't think you had or that mattered. In truth, togetherness has the potential to be one remedy for the many symptoms of depression. It's okay to ask for the help you need.

Going on an anti-inflammatory diet (page 66) can be extremely beneficial if depression has been a lifelong issue. Our gut health and mental well-being are incredibly connected.

PRACTICE: A CALL FOR CONNECTION

More than any other remedy, the need for community and togetherness seems to be often overlooked in how we move through depression, grief, despair, rage, and other difficult emotions. Staying home, in bed, locked away from the world, watching Netflix all day might be a nice thing to do every once in a while, but chances are if you've been stuck in this cycle, you need to reach out to a friend or find a new way to put yourself out there in order to shift your energy and open yourself up to new people and possibilities.

We are social creatures, and part of our self-care involves building a support system (page 35). When we feel seen and validated in our experiences, we feel less alone, and that in itself is enormously healing.

Let's face it: our society doesn't always encourage us to express how we feel openly and with honesty, so it can be difficult to ask for what we need. Consider seeking out a like-minded community or a professional therapist who encourages you to access your emotions, talk through hardships more freely, and find the motivation to be the person you want to be.

Next time you're feeling low, depressed, or stuck, try these acts to cultivate a sense of belonging and care:

→ Call up a friend to vent.

→ Ask your partner for extra support during a particularly trying week, month, or season.

→ Invite a friend to go on a walk in the park, visit a museum, or grab a bite to eat with you.

→ Ride the bus, see a movie by yourself, take yourself out on a solo dinner date, sit in a public place and people-watch—these kinds of activities allow you to be alone while appreciating that you are a part of something bigger.

→ Attend a community function or spiritual group weekly or monthly.

→ Volunteer at a nonprofit organization.

→ Attend a breathwork, meditation, or art class.

HERBS AND FLOWER ESSENCES

Herbs and flower essences can provide emotional resilience, gut healing, and nervous-system support. Focus on restorative, nourishing, aromatic, gently stimulating, and uplifting herbs like:

→ Ashwagandha

→ Black pepper

→ Damiana

→ Garlic

→ Ginger

→ Hawthorn

→ Holy basil/tulsi

→ Mimosa

→ Nettle

→ Oat

→ Reishi

→ Rose

→ Rosemary

→ Skullcap

→ St. John's wort

In addition, stimulating adaptogens like ethically sourced American or Asian ginseng or eleuthero can be added to the mix if you're struggling to have the energy to show up for basic tasks like caring for the kids, preparing meals, or getting to work.

Remember, if there are gut issues, nutrient absorption and chronic inflammation might play into your lack of energy, lethargy, and brain fog. Some favorites that combat depression and digestive distress are

→ Calendula

→ Chamomile

→ Ginger

→ Lemon balm

→ Licorice

→ Marshmallow root

→ Meadowsweet

If you want to work with flower essences for depression, try mustard and olive to start. Mustard is an excellent remedy for sudden episodes of depression that seem to come out of nowhere. When you're unsure of the cause of your sudden moodiness and tend toward gloomy, defeated thoughts, work with mustard. Olive aids us when physical and mental exhaustion plays a role in depression. Our body just can't keep up with the demands we've placed on it, so we collapse.

Lemon Balm (*Melissa officinalis*)

PARTS USED leaf

ENERGETICS slightly warming

Lemon balm is a gleeful addition to any home apothecary. An aromatic mint family plant, lemon balm's fragrant leaves have many healing virtues. Wherever this plant grows, bees are sure to follow. In fact, the genus name, *Melissa*, is the namesake of a nymph who, in Greek mythology, shared the wisdom of bees and the curative uses of their honey. This sweet-scented herb is notable for its calming and uplifting traits that declutter the mind if it is buzzing like a bee. When life feels like too much to handle, reach for lemon balm.

Lemon balm helps us enjoy the simple pleasures of being alive. A gentle mood elevator and heart tonic, lemon balm is sure to put us in good spirits when part of our daily self-care. We all have that well-meaning friend (real talk—maybe this is you) who seems to always be a naysayer, overly focused on all the things that could go wrong, their pessimism or apathy raining down on every possibility. Offer them a spoonful of lemon balm honey or a strong cup of lemon balm infusion to remind them of the possibilities and goodness in life. If you get stuck in a doom-and-gloom mindset, have bouts of seasonal depression, or generally feel moody and dissatisfied, lemon balm can be your new best friend. Lemon balm is also excellent for headaches or muscular pain associated with tension.

In addition, lemon balm can ease abdominal cramping, gas, and bloating and generally supports digestion. For general immune support and to alleviate the tendency to feel mentally and emotional low when sick, add lemon balm to your favorite immune formulas.

WORD TO THE WISE Lemon balm is a great preventative herb for the herpes virus, especially if herpes outbreaks are triggered during times of stress. Add lemon balm to a tincture formula with holy basil/tulsi, licorice, and St. John's wort, and take at the first sign of symptoms. In addition, you can make a lemon balm salve by infusing the plant in the carrier oil of your choice and adding a few drops of lemon balm essential oil. Be sure to apply with a cotton swab or clean finger so as not to spread the virus.

SUGGESTED PREPARATIONS hot Infusion, honey, tincture

FAVORITE PLANT PAIRINGS ginger, elderberry, St. John's wort, rose, damiana

CAUTION Not for use with thyroid medications, as it inhibits the effects of THS (thyroid-stimulating hormone)

Uplift Infusion

For days when you're feeling defeated, exhausted, agitated, in a fog, or otherwise down in the dumps. This infusion can be enjoyed throughout the day to help encourage lightheartedness and calm when all seems heavy and pointless. Try preparing a cup first thing in the morning the next time you wake with a case of the Mondays.

MAKES 4 CUPS

> 3 tablespoons lemon balm
> 2 teaspoons linden leaf
> 2 teaspoons gotu kola
> 5–10 drops of mustard flower essence or essence of choice

NOTE: All herbs should be cut and sifted.

To make the blend, add all ingredients to a small jar, put the lid on, and shake thoroughly to combine. Label the jar with the blend title, ingredients, and the date you made it. Store the blend out of direct sunlight and it will keep for 8–12 months.

When ready to drink Uplift Infusion, use 1 heaping tablespoon of the blend for every 8 ounces of water. For a single serving, add 1 tablespoon to a reusable tea strainer. Alternatively, you can add the blend to a glass jar or French press and brew up to 32 ounces. Bring water to a boil and pour it over the blend and allow to steep for a minimum of 15 minutes. Drink hot or refrigerate and enjoy chilled.

Lemon Balm and Orange Peel Honey

This herbal honey tastes like summer in a jar, and we can all use a helping of that on our hardest days.

MAKES 8-OUNCE JAR

3 tablespoons lemon balm

1 tablespoon orange peel

3–5 slices fresh ginger

I cup local raw honey

See page 229 for instructions on making herbal honey.

Enjoy this honey by the spoonful on cloudy, gray days when you're feeling down; during the long winter months to brighten your mood and strengthen immunity and fight infection; or to replace eating junk food when you're having a sugar craving. Add to tea or enjoy by the spoonful to bring a much-needed smile to your face. This honey is mood-elevating, immune-supportive, and a digestive aid.

NOTE: Children under one year old should not be given honey.

Damiana (*Turnera diffusa*)

PARTS USED leaf

ENERGETICS warming

Damiana is a small shrub native to southwest Texas, Mexico, and parts of Central and South America and has been used by the indigenous peoples of Mexico and Latin America since the time of the Mayan civilization. Damiana is a warming, gently stimulating plant that manages to bring on feelings of giddiness and complete relaxation instantaneously. It loosens tension throughout, empowering bodily awareness and comfort and allowing us to embrace the present. This can be useful for folks who tend to disconnect from their bodies due to physical pain, body shame, or past trauma. Both aromatic and bitter, damiana stimulates the interplay between our nervous and digestive systems, rekindling an awareness of gut intuition, the need for self-preservation, and grounding.

An herb for igniting the life force, damiana can help shift patterns of isolation, bringing us outward and enlivening our senses so that we can find renewed pleasure in connection. It's an indispensable herb for when you find yourself stuck in your head or in a bad mood. Combine with your choice of holy basil/tulsi, ginger, lemon balm, mimosa, or rosemary for mental fatigue, brain fog, or depression. Long-term use will strengthen and restore resiliency to your nervous system and improve your energy and inner fire.

WORD TO THE WISE Damiana brings awareness and circulation to the extremities and pelvis and is considered an aphrodisiac. This herb can be a wonderful addition to self-care practices when sexual vigor is depleted due to chronic stress, depression, fatigue, or anxiety.

SUGGESTED PREPARATIONS tea, elixir, body oil

FAVORITE PLANT PAIRINGS kava, rose, wood betony, hawthorn, rosemary

Enliven Elixir

Feeling stuck, stressed, sunk in? This blend will support you in shifting out of these states. If you experience low spirits, worry, and anxiety, this can be a lovely medicine to bring comfort and ease to body and mind.

MAKES 3 CUPS

4 cups water

4 tablespoons damiana

3 tablespoons holy basil/tulsi

3 tablespoons hawthorn berry

2 tablespoons rose petals

1 tablespoon kava

1 cup sweetener of choice—local raw honey or
    unrefined cane sugar usually works best

½–1 cup alcohol of choice

OPTIONAL: 5–10 drops flower essence of choice before bottling

See page 227 for instructions on making an elixir.

Take up to a tablespoon of elixir twice daily to support yourself through heartbreak, grief, or depression. Enliven Elixir can be added to sparkling or filtered water, a cup of tea, or taken by a dropper straight in the mouth. When using a dropper, 3–4 dropperfuls will equal about 1 teaspoon. Store syrup in the refrigerator and it will last for up to 6 months.

Banish the Blues Tincture

A daily formula that will support you through depression, melancholy, brain fog, fatigue, and overwhelming stress.

MAKES 4-OUNCE (120 ML) BOTTLE

40 milliliters damiana alcohol extract

30 milliliters holy basil/tulsi alcohol extract

20 milliliters lemon balm alcohol extract

10 milliliters calendula alcohol extract

10 milliliters rosemary alcohol extract

OPTIONAL: 5–10 drops flower essence of choice

See page 235 for instructions on making a tincture.

Take 1–2 dropperfuls twice daily for an extended period—minimum 4–6 weeks—to help with overall feelings of lethargy, exhaustion, mental fatigue, mild depression, and brain fog. This tincture can be added to a few inches of drinking water, added to a smoothie or juice, or put directly in the mouth.

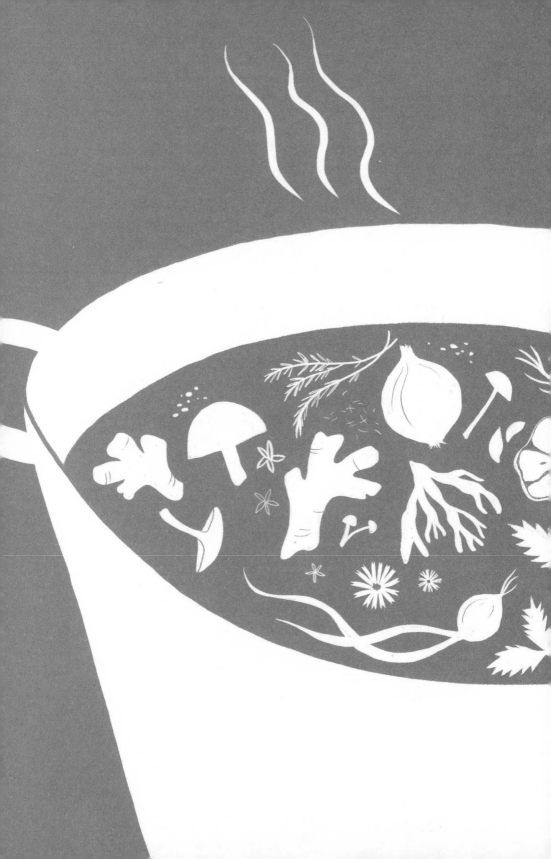

Tending to Your Immunity

8

THE IMMUNE SYSTEM'S ROLE is to protect us from infection and unwelcome microorganisms. It is our body's defense system, and it is constantly adapting to our social, chemical, and biological needs and demands. A complex, highly intelligent, interconnected network of cells, tissues, and organs, the immune system is anywhere and everywhere in the body, from your skin and mouth to your GI tract and blood; it's ready to snap into action. Therefore, keeping your immune system functioning in tip-top shape is of utmost importance in maintaining the health and functioning of all the other systems of the body. Diet and lifestyle, in tandem with taking immune-modulating and strengthening herbs on a daily basis, can keep your entire being healthy and happy.

The immune system functions by identifying self from nonself. The immune system's ability to correctly discern between self and nonself is honed and remembered as we move through life and encounter various pathogens. The resulting knowledge falls into two categories: innate immunity and adaptive immunity. We are born with innate immunity, which is inherited from our parents. This immunity is your first line of nonspecific defense and includes the external barriers of the body like the skin and the mucus membranes of the mouth, throat, and GI tract. This type of immunity is more effective in the short term and needs support. Adaptive, or acquired, immunity develops as we grow and age, storing a library of antibodies to different germs or pathogens. These antibodies come to our aid when our innate immunity doesn't hold up.

These types of immunities work in unison to keep us well. Herbal medicine works to fortify both types: you can work with herbs daily as preventative medicine as well as use them to boost the efficiency of your immune system in case, for example, you catch a virus.

YOUR IMMUNITY TOOLKIT

FLUIDS

Staying hydrated is crucial to maintaining your immune system. Fluids protect your mucous membranes, keeping them moist and resilient while replenishing electrolytes and keeping germs and toxins flushed and moving out of your body. Take special care to make sure you're getting the fluids you need every day. This includes sipping water throughout the day in addition to herbal infusions and broth when you start to feel under the weather.

MEDICINAL MUSHROOMS

Medicinal mushrooms such as reishi, turkey tail, shiitake, lion's mane, cordyceps, and maitake prime and strengthen the immune system so that over time your immune cells become smarter at fending off pathogens. This can be especially beneficial with allergies and when the immune system becomes unnecessarily overactive. Many culinary mushrooms like shiitake and maitake can be added to stir-fries and soups, while woody, tougher mushrooms like reishi and turkey tail will need to be simmered for a few hours and made into broths, teas, or decoctions for tinctures. Each medicinal mushroom has its own specific qualities beyond the immune system, so seek out further information (see resources, page 241).

Do some research and find out which mushrooms grow in your region and which ones are best for you. Support local mushroom growers and medicine-makers who harvest mushrooms sustainably, with respect for the fungi. As medicinal mushrooms have become more popular, overharvesting and irresponsible practices can devastate an ecosystem that depends on these fungi while flooding the market with mushrooms that aren't as medicinally potent.

FERMENTED AND PUNGENT FOODS

Fermented foods like sauerkraut, kimchi, yogurt, miso, and kefir provide you with a daily dose of beneficial bacteria. Good bacteria such as lactobacillus and bifidobacterium help fight off pathogens and bad bacteria that can play into poor health, weakened immunity, gut and skin complaints, mood-related issues, and inflammation.

> Herbal medicine works to fortify both types: you can work with herbs daily as preventative medicine as well as use them to boost the efficiency of your immune system in case, for example, you catch a virus.

Pungent foods like onions, garlic, ginger, horseradish, wasabi, black pepper, and spicy chili peppers can do wonders for a sluggish or cold body, an unrelenting runny nose, congestion, or a wet cough. These foods bring warmth and circulation to the whole body while more specifically enhancing digestion, opening your airways, and encouraging mucus flow that helps get germs out of the body. In addition, these foods—along with pungent herbs like clove, oregano, rosemary, and thyme—are antimicrobial.

HEALTHY FATS

Much like staying hydrated, healthy fats also help lubricate inside and out. Notably, healthy fats support immune-cell functioning and assist the nervous system. If you feel like you drink plenty of water but still experience symptoms like dry skin, inflammation, a constant tickle in the throat, dry sinuses, constipation, or a frayed nervous system, healthy fats give you the buffer your body needs. Your entire body requires healthy fats to function properly, so seek out fatty fish like wild salmon, herring, or sardines (or a high-quality fishoil supplement); quality oils such as olive; and nuts and seeds.

Strengthening and Modulating Immunity

A resilient, balanced immune system is one of the best things any of us can ask for. When the immune system is weak or deficient, you may get sick more often than your loved ones or never fully recover from certain symptoms, such as a sinus infection that lingers for months. Immunity on overdrive happens when your immune response becomes hyper-reactive to a real or perceived pathogen, such as when we experience allergies or autoimmune disorders.

Autoimmune issues like lupus or arthritis happen when the body can't tell self from nonself and begins attacking healthy cells, causing allergies, chronic low-level inflammation, or other complaints, which over time can lead to more severe issues like cancer or cardiovascular disease. Whether weakened or on overdrive, what the immune system needs is balancing. Medicinal herbs, along with diet and lifestyle shifts, help us fine-tune our immunity, so it works for us and not against us.

LIFESTYLE

When it comes to strengthening your immune system, you'll want to start with evaluating how stressed you are. The nervous system and the immune system are entwined, and research shows that stress can have a catastrophic impact on the resiliency of the immune system, especially the regulation of the inflammation response. Take some time to revisit chapters 5 and 6 and consider implementing such practices as breathwork (page 109), mindfulness meditation, and daily exercise to help relieve stress and boost immune function.

Preventative care should focus on much of what was discussed in chapters 3, 4, and 5 concerning how to use herbs and various practices to support digestion, manage stress, and nourish vitality. In addition to taking care of your mental health, strong immunity depends on staying hydrated, eating a healthy diet with lots of colorful fruits and vegetables, getting a good night's sleep, and spending time with community and loved ones.

When we do get sick, it isn't about suppressing or covering up symptoms; it's about contemplating the mechanisms at play (for example, a runny nose, a cough, a fever) and working with herbs that complement how our body wants to heal. For example, a fever is your body trying to heat up to kill the infecting organism. So when you suppress a fever, you're inadvertently halting your body's self-defense. So, drinking a strong, hot infusion of elderflower, hyssop, and peppermint can help encourage and then break a fever.

PRACTICE: MAKING BROTH AT HOME

Broth-making can be a wonderful weekly or monthly practice that helps fortify your whole body. It's a simple, relaxing kitchen activity you can do while listening to music, a podcast, or an audio book. Broth builds and repairs your digestive and immune systems, plus it is full of nutrients that benefit your entire being. You can make broth with chicken or beef bones, tons of mushrooms and veggies, or both. It's really up to you. Both are full of nourishing vitamins and minerals, bringing warmth and healing to your gut and fortifying your nervous and immune systems. Making broth is a terrific fall and winter practice, when your body craves hearty, warming soups. The best part: once you make a batch, you can store it in the freezer and have it on hand for months to come! My favorite is to pour room-temperate broth into ice cube trays so that you can use a little at a time. Add a cube when you're cooking up veggies or rice.

There are so many versions of broth you can make.

For an immune-boosting veggie option, add a roughly chopped knob or two of fresh ginger, a few pieces of dried reishi, a cup of dried shiitakes, an onion cut in quarters, a handful of roughly cut celery or leeks, 5–8 whole garlic cloves cut in half, and a ½ cup of nettle leaf and sprigs of fresh thyme to a stockpot filled with 8–10 cups of water. This makes an immune-strengthening, nourishing broth that can be sipped or used as a base for soup.

HERBS AND FLOWER ESSENCES

Herbs that build and modulate the immune system should be taken regularly in the form of infusions, tinctures, and foods like medicinal broths, stir-fries, and any other recipes you can dream up. These modulating herbs help prevent illnesses like the common cold and flu and can be beneficial for addressing a variety of complaints like asthma, allergies, autoimmune disorders, and even for cancer care.

If you tend to feel congested, fatigued, and always a little sick with something, invest in a few immune-modulating and strengthening herbs to take daily, like ashwagandha, astragalus, holy basil/tulsi, licorice, reishi, and shiitake.

Reishi *(Ganoderma lucidum)*

PARTS USED fruiting body

ENERGETICS slightly warming, neutral

A true tonic herb, reishi builds us up so we can live a long and fulfilling life. Known as the mushroom of immortality, this adaptogen nourishes and balances many body systems simultaneously. Renowned for its ability to increase the resiliency of the immune system, reishi also calms and nourishes the heart, offers emotional balance, improves cognitive function, protects the liver, and modulates an overactive stress response. In an age of stress and anxiety, reishi soothes and strengthens the nervous system and adrenals. A fortifying herb, this mushroom is best suited for long-term daily use. Strive to cultivate a relationship with this ancient medicine instead of expecting overnight results.

If you or a loved one seems to always be getting sick or dealing with nervous exhaustion, insomnia, or chronic illness or pain, work with reishi to restore wellness. Reishi is also an excellent ally for those working through any kind of trauma, loss, or depression, or feel disconnected and depleted. It is gentle enough to be taken by most anyone.

WORD TO THE WISE Recognizing the cycles of your body based on seasonal shifts can offer helpful cues. If you tend to suffer from seasonal allergies, begin to take reishi in the weeks leading up to when you usually start to experience symptoms. If the winter months have you plagued with one cold after another, start incorporating reishi into your self-care in the autumn.

SUGGESTED PREPARATIONS broth, decoction, tincture

FAVORITE PLANT PAIRINGS ginger, shiitake mushrooms, astragalus, rose, skullcap

Immune Upkeep Tincture

An immune-strengthening companion to help keep your immune system in tip-top shape. Use this formula in the month or two leading up to allergy season or for daily immune maintenance during the winter months.

MAKES 4-OUNCE (120 ML) BOTTLE

40 milliliters reishi alcohol extract
20 milliliters astragalus alcohol extract
20 milliliters calendula alcohol extract
20 milliliters lemon balm alcohol extract
10 milliliters ginger alcohol extract
10 milliliters nettle alcohol extract

See page 235 for instructions on making a tincture.

Take 1–2 dropperfuls twice daily for an extended period—minimum 4–6 weeks—to help strengthen and balance the immune system and for lymph support, healthy digestion, and to ward off allergies. This tincture can be added to a few inches of drinking water, added to a smoothie or juice, or put directly in the mouth.

Love Your Lymph

Considering how important the lymphatic system is to the underlying function of not only your immune system but your entire body, it's surprising that lymphatic herbs and lymphatic health in general aren't talked about more. White blood cells are stored and transported by the lymphatic system, which includes the lymph nodes (found in places like under the jawline, armpits, and groin), thymus, bone marrow, spleen, tonsils, appendix, and Peyer's patches in the small intestine.

The lymphatic system helps detoxify the body by cleaning up waste and ushering it out by way of the circulatory system. It also transports infection-fighting white blood cells, which spring into action when you start to get sick. You may have experienced this happening when you start feeling under the weather and your neck feels swollen and tender. Those are your lymph nodes hard at work, fending off an infection.

Unlike the circulatory system, where the heart pumps and moves blood and oxygen throughout the body, the lymphatic system relies on the movement of muscles throughout the day to help keep things flowing like a healthy stream of water. Sedentary lifestyles—sitting for long hours at work and lack of exercise—can cause stagnation in the lymph, which can result in imbalances both physical and emotional.

Any complaint with a chronic inflammation or a skin component (autoimmunity, cold or flu, arthritis, swollen lymph glands, cancer, eczema, acne, chronic asthma), or issues like sluggish menstruation, water retention, and uterine fibroids, or even feeling emotionally stuck, aimless, or repressed will benefit from the addition of herbs for lymph health, along with lymph-supportive practices like regular exercise or stretching, body oiling, dry brushing, and lymph massage.

LIFESTYLE

Daily exercise and an active lifestyle go a long way in supporting your lymph. Evening walks, any kind of rigorous exercise (hitting the gym, doing some jumping jacks, or jogging up and down the stairs at work), yoga (especially inversions) will all be beneficial.

In addition, getting regular massages, giving yourself weekly rubdowns with herbal oils, or practicing dry brushing are all supportive of lymph health. Lastly, stay hydrated, drink herbal infusions with nutritive herbs and lymph movers, and focus on eating lots of raw and cooked veggies.

PRACTICE: DRY BRUSHING

Dry brushing is an integral part of the Ayurvedic healing tradition of India. This practice is recommended for sluggishness of body and mind. Its benefits include giving your skin a thorough exfoliation, removing dry and dead skin, and stimulating your circulation and lymphatic drainage.

In dry brushing, the skin is typically brushed toward the heart, starting at the feet. As you move up your body, including your arms, abdomen, and parts of your back that you can reach, you continue to brush toward your heart. Use firm, small strokes on longer limbs like arms and legs and work in a circular motion around joints like the ankles, knees, hips, elbows, and shoulders. All you'll need is a natural-bristle brush, which can be found at most natural grocery stores or online. Find a firmness that works for you; the point isn't to rub your skin raw, but a little redness isn't a bad thing either. Make sure your skin is completely dry before doing this. Ideally, you would do this once or twice a week as an invigorating morning routine before hopping in the shower and starting your day. The entire process takes five to ten minutes.

HERBS AND FLOWER ESSENCES

The nice thing about herbs with an affinity for the lymphatic system is that we end up supporting our entire being when we ingest them. Many of these herbs work really well for skin issues like eczema and acne. These herbs come to our aid when we are starting to get sick and have swollen lymph nodes and need to make sure the immune system is ready to fight infection. In addition, these herbs cleanse the blood and help with general detoxification and liver support. Work with herbs known as lymph movers—calendula, cleavers, echinacea, red root, violet—to support your lymph health.

Calendula and violet are my favorites when combined in a lymph-supporting body oil. Try adding the flowers to teas, salads, or broths. Violet and dandelion flower syrup in the spring is a great lymph-lovin' treat. Calendula tea or tincture should definitely be used if there is a gut-related issue or an underlying digestive complaint. Chickweed and violet leaf are excellent added to salads; and cleavers, chickweed, and nettle make a wonderful pesto. You will find that many detoxification and lymph herbs are considered weeds, so keep a lookout in your neighborhood. Just make sure the surrounding area is clean and free of nasty sprays and pesticides.

Cleavers (*Galíum aparíne*)

PARTS USED aerial parts

ENERGETICS cool, moist

A delightful spring tonic that grows throughout North America and Europe, cleavers is a common weed that can be found in most vacant lots and fields, and even on city sidewalks. You may have already met this sticky companion, since mature cleavers have a tendency to cling to other plants and humans alike, a tactic that helps this plant spread its seed. Much like dandelion, cleavers is some of the first growth after the long winter months, and its medicine is much needed after the stagnation and excesses that occur during those times of sedation and heavy meals.

A cooling, detoxifying plant, cleavers is an ideal remedy for swollen lymph glands, including the tonsils as well as glands in the armpits, breasts, and groin. For this, a topical and/or internal application can be used in tandem at the first sign of swollen glands or, in the case of more long-standing complaints, as a daily routine to support the lymphatic and immune systems.

Lightly massage herb-infused cleavers oil on the swollen area, make a cleavers-infused vinegar to dress salads, and take cleavers internally as a tincture or infusion.

WORD TO THE WISE Cleavers is a nonirritating diuretic that increases the flow of urine and further supports the body's ability to cleanse. Have cleavers on hand if you suffer from urinary or bladder complaints, especially UTIs with a hot, burning sensation. Try a quart of marshmallow root and cleavers cold infusion and drink daily until symptoms subside. Since cleavers supports detoxification of your body by way of the kidneys and lymph, consider working with cleavers if you are troubled with skin conditions like psoriasis, eczema, or chronic acne.

SUGGESTED PREPARATIONS infusion, herbal vinegar, herbal oil

FAVORITE PLANT PAIRINGS calendula, violet, red root, nettle

Lymph Love Massage Oil

This oil is an indispensable ally for anyone with chronic immunity issues, poor circulation, or sluggishness. Herbs like cleavers, calendula, and violet unite to improve lymph circulation and detoxify the body while improving the immune system's defense. Massage your whole body or prioritize the area around your armpits and chest while checking for lumps.

MAKES 8-OUNCE JAR

> 3 tablespoons cleavers
> 2 tablespoons calendula
> 1 tablespoon violet leaf and/or flower
> 1 cup carrier oil(s) of choice (try one or a combination of organic, cold-pressed, unrefined almond, apricot kernel, olive, and sesame)

See page 237 for instructions on making herbal oil.

To use, massage a quarter-sized amount into hands and massage on clean skin, prioritizing areas that have a higher concentration of lymph, like around the armpits and upper chest as this can be a daily or weekly preventative ritual to support chest health and to stay aware of any changes your body makes. In addition, this oil can be used daily to moisturize your whole body while gaining the added benefits of improving lymph health. Start at your feet and move your hands upward, massaging the oil into your legs, improving the circulation as you go.

If you start to get sick and notice your lymph nodes swelling under your jaw, add a few drops to your fingertips and massage the oil into your neck, starting at your jawline and moving downward to your collarbones. This will encourage healthy lymph drainage and boost immunity.

Lung, Throat, and Sinus Care

Infection manifests in all of us differently, and for those who are prone to respiratory complaints like sinus infections, asthma, sore throats, and coughs, it can make a huge difference to have certain herbs ready on the defense. This system, principally the lungs, is an incredibly important vital organ with the life-sustaining task of balancing oxygen and carbon dioxide levels in our body.

Fortunately, herbs and natural therapies can be extremely helpful for more serious problems like chronic lung and sinus complaints, as well as everyday respiratory trouble you might encounter. Medicinal herbs complement any medical care you might already be receiving from a doctor, so there's no need to pick and choose. But if you are someone who wants to be less reliant on your inhaler or medication, herbal allies and lifestyle shifts can truly change your relationship with your respiratory system, healing imbalances and minimizing the need for drugs.

LIFESTYLE

When it comes to chronic issues like asthma, that sinus infection you never seem to fully shake, or seasonal allergies that happen like clockwork, lifestyle shifts and self-care practices can come in handy, empowering you and offering noticeable relief.

Preventative practices like stress management with breathing exercises, plenty of rest, and a good night's sleep are paramount. Do your best to keep away from situations or substances that irritate the respiratory system. Supporting your immune and respiratory systems with lots of aromatic, medicinally potent herbs and foods is another big one.

If you notice any food sensitivities, remove the problem foods altogether or, at the very least, limit them to an occasional treat. You may wish to go on an anti-inflammatory diet (page 66) to rebuild and repair your entire body. If sinus infections, congestion in the lungs, or a stuffy or runny nose or allergies are chronic issues, you should consider the amount of dairy you eat and completely remove all dairy whenever you are having an infection, attack, or are generally sick. Dairy creates mucus and will only worsen the problem. Always consider how you can best work with your body instead of against it.

PRACTICE: HERBAL STEAMS

Oftentimes, herbal steams get left out of the healing conversation compared to tinctures, teas, and syrups, or they are talked about solely for beautification and skin health. But when I start to feel an infection taking hold in my upper respiratory system, an herbal face steam is my first and most trusted defense. Often, the first signs of the cold or flu are an opportunity, an invitation even, for you to prioritize your health and slow down. Doing so with yummy syrups and relaxing facial steams makes the stress of getting sick feel a little more like an excuse to pamper yourself.

Steam opens pores, improves circulation, and relaxes inflamed sinuses while promoting healthy airways. Breathing in the steam of whole, dried, or fresh plants—some of my personal favorites are oregano, peppermint, pine, rosemary, and thyme—further aid the steam by loosening congestion, targeting the infection and keeping it from moving or settling into the lungs. Any aromatic kitchen herb will do as they are wonderful remedies for respiratory ailments due to their fierce antimicrobial compounds.

In a small pot, bring a few inches of water to a simmer and add the herb(s) of your choice. Turn the heat off and, with a towel over your head, hover over the pot for 5–10 minutes and breathe deeply. Repeat every few hours to help kick a sinus infection or keep congestion from turning into a sore throat or lung complaint.

PRACTICE: HOLY SMOKE

The burning of herbs and resins is an ancient and sacred practice that spans continents and cultures. As long as there has been fire, there has been the burning of herbs to protect, cleanse, dispel bad spirits, or set intention for ceremony. The fascinating thing is, all of these herbs that are burned for more magical, energetic, or spiritual uses are also incredible at warding off pathogens and protecting the immune system.

As we breathe in the potently medicinal aromatics of plants like cedar, frankincense, garden sage, juniper, mugwort, myrrh, pine, or rosemary, we ward off unwanted infection, safeguarding our immunity and strengthening our physical barrier. You can do this at home by burning incense made from the herbs listed here, by burning dried herbs or resins in a small dish, or by carefully holding a small bundle of dried herbs in your hand and wafting the smoke around your room. Keep some clippings from your holiday tree or wreath and burn those for months to come.

Respect Plants and People

If you are wanting to work with spiritually potent herbs for burning or ingestion, it's critical that you research your own ancestry and not appropriate and exploit the spiritual and culturally significant plants of indigenous peoples. Using plants from your ancestry connects you with those who came before you and strengthens the work you're doing. If the spiritual or magical uses of medicinal herbs interests you, that's great! Just take some time to learn about how to be in right relationship with your ancestral ways and respect the plants and people of other traditions. Try to refrain from working with herbs like palo santo (*Bursera graveolens*) and white sage (*Salvia apiana*), two herbs burned and used for their aromatic smoke, as both run the risk of overharvesting due to rising commercial demand and lack of habitat due to global warming and industry.

In California, where white sage is a native species, tribes in the region have been working with and stewarding this plant for hundreds of years. They have repeatedly asked that nonindigenous people not wildcraft or sell it, as it is a sacred ceremonial plant in their traditions. White sage and palo santo are both critically threated plant species that require practitioners and customers alike to take a stand. Both plants have been sold on the market for spiritual cleansing and to purify spaces, but how a plant is picked, processed, and sold has an enormous impact on its potency—whether for spiritual or medicinal means.

If you are adamant about working with white sage, grow your own or buy directly from someone who cultivates it instead of wildcrafting. And under no circumstance should you be using the essential oils of these plants, as this is wholly unsustainable. Hundreds and sometimes thousands of pounds of plant material are needed to produce just one gallon of essential oil.

HERBS AND FLOWER ESSENCES

Herbs can both treat and manage respiratory issues. When dealing with an infection in your lungs, throat, or sinuses, work with herbs that are aromatic, inflammation-reducing, and antimicrobial to help ward off the infection.

When working with herbs, you can do a number of things to improve your health and balance longstanding issues. Herbal medicine can assist by

→ opening airways and improving the utilization of oxygen (elecampane, mullein, thyme)

→ soothing irritation and dry cough (bee balm, elderberry, garden sage, holy basil/tulsi, honey, licorice, marshmallow, mullein, mint)

→ reducing histamine and thinning mucus in sinuses (goldenrod, nettle)

→ fighting infection and inflammation (elecampane, garden sage, garlic, ginger, propolis, rosemary, sea salt, thyme)

→ draining sinuses and moving nasal and lung congestion (angelica, elecampane, ginger, goldenrod, horseradish, nettle, thyme)

→ strengthening and repairing the immune and respiratory systems (astragalus, holy basil/tulsi, licorice, reishi)

As you can see, there is a wide variety of herbs that are supportive, so pick a few that grow abundantly near you and work with those consistently.

Lymphatic support is crucial when combating illness, so incorporating calendula, cleavers, or red root into a tincture blend is a great way to go. At the first sign of a sore or scratchy throat, congested sinuses, or other personal signals that your body might be catching something, immediately start taking immune-stimulating and lymphatic moving herbs like echinacea, which doesn't so much kill the infection as it boosts immunity into action. A tincture of cleavers, echinacea, lemon balm, and licorice is a personal favorite, though if you tend to have a wet cough or lots of congestion and mucus, replace the licorice with elecampane, which thins mucus while soothing a cough.

An elderberry, goldenrod, and nettle tincture is excellent support at the onset of seasonal allergies, sinus congestion, and mucus buildup. Try doing an herbal stream with aromatic herbs that will help loosen congestion and reduce inflammation (page 175). Foods like citrus, garlic, horseradish, onions, and spicy peppers can be added to food or combined and added to apple cider vinegar. Take a look at the seasonal wellness chart (pages 30–31) for more remedies.

Culinary Herbs
to the Rescue

For beginners to herbal medicine, the task of creating a home apothecary can seem a bit daunting, not to mention pricey. Good news: many of the herbs you can find at your local grocery store like garlic, ginger, onion, oregano, rosemary, sage, and thyme are incredibly medicinal. Not only are these more familiar kitchen herbs a great place to start, but it can also be empowering to learn the curative ways of something you have in your pantry at this very moment. Working with common culinary herbs to make delicious meals, sinus-cleansing herbal steams, throat-soothing honeys, immune-boosting broths, infection-fighting tinctures, and aromatic teas can remind you that healing is always within reach and doesn't require fancy herbs or lots of money.

Oregano, rosemary, sage, and thyme are all mint family plants that offer a powerhouse of medicine. They are germ-fighting and immune-boosting, with an affinity for the lungs and sinuses, making them perfect for when you wake up with a tingling in your throat or a runny or stuffy nose. Add these to your herbal steam (page 175) and you'll stop illness in its tracks.

Elecampane (*Inula helenium*)

PARTS USED root

ENERGETICS warming, drying

Modern herbalists lean heavily on this dependable sunflower family plant for all manner of respiratory issues. An outstanding expectorant and stimulating ally, the root of elecampane is best suited for stubborn coughs with stuck mucus and phlegm. If you are prone to bronchitis, sinusitis, asthma, wet coughs, or general congestion made worse by damp and cold, elecampane will surely be a welcome addition to your home apothecary. Elecampane also has a mild effect on the lymphatic tissue of the body and is useful for swollen glands in the throat.

A bitter, aromatic, inulin-rich plant, elecampane excels at supporting healthy gut bacteria and overall digestive health when consumed as an herbal infusion or tincture. Inulin is a soluble fiber found in the roots of many medicinal plants like chicory, burdock, and dandelion, as well as in foods like artichokes, asparagus, and onions. Inulin is a prebiotic, feeding healthy gut bacteria. When you have a functioning digestive system, proper nutrient absorption, and happy gut flora, your immune system will work more efficiently. The bitter quality of elecampane tones the digestive tract, regulates blood sugar, supports appetite, and assists with digestion.

WORD TO THE WISE In Traditional Chinese Medicine, grief is thought to be stored in the lungs. If you are grief-stricken with heartbreak or homesickness, add a respiratory herb like elecampane in addition to heart herbs like hawthorn and rose to your self-care routine.

SUGGESTED PREPARATIONS honey, syrup, tincture

FAVORITE PLANT PAIRINGS ginger, thyme, elderberry, orange peel

Elecampane and Thyme Honey

The aromatic, antimicrobial, immune-boosting trio of orange peel, elecampane, and thyme, especially when combined with the therapeutics of raw honey and ginger, makes a great addition to any home apothecary. This honey fights any respiratory infection while coating and soothing a sore throat.

MAKES 8-OUNCE JAR

2 tablespoons elecampane
1 tablespoon orange peel
1 tablespoon thyme
A few slices of fresh ginger
1 cup local raw honey

See page 229 for instructions on making herbal honey.

Enjoy this honey by the spoonful to strengthen immunity and fight infection or to replace eating junk food when you're having a sugar craving. Add to tea or enjoy a spoonful whenever you'd like a little sweetness. This honey supports the immune and respiratory systems while fighting off viral and bacterial infections, plus it's a digestive aid.

NOTE: Children under one year old should not be given honey.

Respiratory Aid Tincture

When you have a wet cough with phlegm, this is the formula for you.

MAKES 2-OUNCE (60 ML) BOTTLE

20 milliliters elecampane alcohol extract

20 milliliters thyme alcohol extract

10 milliliters calendula alcohol extract

10 milliliters rosemary alcohol extract

See page 235 for instructions on making a tincture.

Take 1–2 dropperfuls twice daily for an extended period—minimum 2–4 weeks—to help with chronic cough or a longstanding respiratory infection. In a pinch, for more acute situations such as at the first sign of a cough or sinus infection, take 2–4 dropperfuls every few hours until symptoms start to subside. This tincture can be added to a few inches of drinking water, added to a smoothie or juice, or put directly in the mouth.

Viral Infections

We coexist in this world with viruses, bacteria, and fungi. These microorganisms support a healthy functioning gut, are essential in the fermentation process that gives us bread and beer, are the delicious mushrooms you add to your pizza or take medicinally, and can even be used in the treatment of major diseases. And this is only a few of the amazing ways bacteria, fungi, and viruses play a positive role in our lives.

Sometimes, as we know, these microorganisms can be a little less amazing and a lot more troublesome. Known as pathogens or germs, these microorganisms can cause mild to severe illness and even death. Certain strains can be downright dangerous and extremely contagious.

One of the best ways to ward off the negative effects of germs and infectious disease while enjoying the benefits of all the positives these organisms provide is to maintain proper hygiene, like washing your hands, and work with medicinal herbs on a daily basis. Certain herbs have the potential to strengthen your immune system over time, while herbs known as antimicrobials fight off germs without completely destroying the bacteria, fungi, and viruses that live inside you in a mutually symbiotic way.

Throughout this section we'll explore the herbal allies and practices to ward off and combat viral infections like the common cold, flu, and herpes simplex virus. Whether it's for prevention or support after you've gotten sick or are in the midst of an outbreak, herbal medicine really shines when fighting off viral complaints. Although many of the herbs highlighted—like elderberry, lemon balm, and licorice—are prized for their antiviral abilities, they are also good antimicrobials and can be used for many bacterial or fungal complaints. An antimicrobial is any plant or medicine that wards off a wide spectrum of harmful bacteria, fungi, and viruses. Many of the herbs in this chapter, as well as in other parts of this book, are powerful antimicrobials, especially herbs that are either aromatic and/or bitter tasting like:

- → Angelica
- → Bee balm
- → Calendula
- → Cloves
- → Elecampane
- → Evergreens (pine, juniper, and spruce)
- → Garlic
- → Ginger
- → Hyssop
- → Lemon balm
- → Mint (peppermint, catnip, spearmint)
- → Mugwort

- → Oregano
- → Oregon grape root
- → Rosemary
- → Sage

- → Spilanthes
- → Thyme
- → Yarrow

TREATING COMMON COLD, FLU, AND HERPES

Some virus-caused diseases include the common cold, flu, warts (all types, genital or otherwise, are caused by various strains of human papillomavirus, or HPV), AIDS, SARS, herpes simplex 1 and 2, and chickenpox. Dealing with viral infections means either getting vaccinated to prevent them in the first place, as with vaccinations against HPV, polio, or the measles; or consistent upkeep with herbs, diet, and life-style in cases like herpes simplex, colds, and flu.

For the most part, once you catch a virus like chickenpox, the common cold, or the flu, your main goal is to boost your immunity so that it can do the best job possible while easing the symptoms. Viral infection symptoms vary depending on the virus and the constitution of the person infected, though the recommended herbal care will be the same in terms of immune-modulating and stimulating medicinal plants in addition to antimicrobial, and specifically antiviral, herbs. The common cold, flu, and herpes simplex 1 and 2 are highlighted in this book, though all viral infections can be combated with these practices and herbal considerations in mind.

The flu and the common cold are both respiratory illnesses, but they are caused by different viruses. These two illnesses have similar symptoms, making it difficult to tell them apart. In general, the flu is worse and more intense than the common cold. While the general symptoms can occur in both the common cold and the flu, the onset (abrupt versus gradual) and the severity of symptoms are a great way to tell the difference. The abrupt onset of symptoms like fatigue or general weakness, fever, chills, body aches, and headache are much more common in the flu than with a cold. If you wake up one morning and can barely move, feel like you've been run over by a truck, and have a fever and chills, it's the flu. The gradual onset of symptoms like a sore throat, a runny or stuffy nose, lung congestion, and a cough is more likely the common cold.

Herpes simplex is actually two viruses: herpes simplex type 1 (HSV-1) and herpes simplex type 2 (HSV-2). According to the World Health Organization, 3.7

billion people under the age of fifty have HSV-1—that's 67 percent of the world's population. And one in six Americans between the ages of fourteen and forty-nine have HSV-2. So, herpes simplex 1 and 2 are increasingly common infections, but they are relatively easy to treat, especially with the support of medicinal herbs, along with diet and lifestyle shifts that you'll use throughout your life. Although herpes simplex does not have a cure, it doesn't have to disrupt your relationships, and given how widespread these conditions are, there's certainly no reason to feel ashamed.

Herpes simplex type 1 is transmitted through oral secretions or sores on the skin, usually around the lips, and can be spread by kissing or sharing objects such as toothbrushes, beverages, or eating utensils. An HSV-1 outbreak is commonly referred to as a *cold sore* or a *fever blister* and is different from a canker sore. Canker sores occur only on the inside of the mouth, are not contagious, and are usually caused by a poor, overly acidic diet that irritates the mouth. Canker sores are not viruses like herpes simplex. Occasionally, HSV-1 can cause genital sores, usually transmitted through oral sex.

An HSV-2 outbreak is known as *genital herpes* and is different than genital warts, which are caused by a different virus. In general, a person is most at risk of getting HSV-2 as a result of sexual contact with someone who has the virus. The risk, of course, is much higher if one partner is having an outbreak, though it is possible to get infected with herpes simplex 1 and 2 anytime. So if you or a loved one is having an outbreak, whether it be cold sores (HSV-1) or genital herpes (HSV-2), it's best to momentarily hit the pause button on kissing, oral sex, penetrative sex, and the sharing of utensils or other objects that come in contact with the mouth or genitals.

Working with herbal remedies and managing your stress levels can offer huge relief for those with herpes simplex 1 and 2. Oftentimes you can stay on top of your stress and immune health with herbal tonics that support the nervous and immune systems. Diet also plays a role in causing an outbreak, so pay attention to food triggers. The herpes virus needs arginine, an amino acid, to grow, so consider limiting or avoiding foods high in arginine such as nuts (especially peanuts), chocolate, soy, breakfast cereals, etc.

Learn to identify the beginnings of an outbreak: tingles, itching, swelling, and mild cold symptoms (fatigue, low fever, etc.). You may also want to supplement with lysine, an amino acid that helps support your immune system and is known to help prevent and treat cold sores. It can be taken daily, while a higher dose should be taken during an outbreak. Herbalist Rosemary Gladstar recommends 500 milligrams three times daily at the first sign of an outbreak.

What about Antibiotics?

It's important to know that antibiotics do nothing for viral infections because viruses are not bacteria. Many doctors feel their patients' expectations that they must come to their aid, so they might prescribe antibiotics in the case of viral infection as a courtesy placebo, without explaining that the antibiotics won't do anything. Prescribing something, even if it does nothing but wipe out healthy gut bacteria as antibiotics do, gives their patients the illusion of support while in reality their bodies have to fight off the virus unsupported by conventional medicine. An additional downside is that with the overprescription of antibiotics, there is a rise of drug-resistant microorganisms. This makes a growing number of infections, both viral and bacterial, harder to treat with drugs and conventional medicine.

Medicinal herbs and home remedies really shine when it comes to preventing and fighting viral infections like the common cold and flu, and they do help decrease the occurrence of outbreaks for those with herpes simplex 1 or 2. These herbs boost and strengthen immunity, so they're far more effective and can ease the discomfort and duration of an illness, all without depleting healthy gut bacteria or suppressing symptoms that are actually useful to your body.

LIFESTYLE

Rest and sleep are critical all the time, but especially so when you're starting to come down with something. Check out the practices from chapter 6 to help you embrace rest and relaxation and ensure a good night's sleep. Take getting sick as an invitation to slow down, and resist the urge to power through or ignore your body. Of course, we all have certain responsibilities that we can't just shrug off, but asking for extra support and rescheduling certain nonessential tasks until you're well can make a big difference. Lie in bed as much as you want, catch up on reading, take a bath or do a foot soak, watch movies, leisurely drink tea. Be sure to remove processed foods, sugar, dairy, and any other foods that you notice make your symptoms worse. Begin eating more fermented foods, warming herbs and spices, and broths.

When it comes to viral infections, a poor diet can stress the system, so make healthy eating a priority. Focus on dark leafy greens, healthy fats, fruits and veggies, nuts and seeds (for example: flax, chia, cashews, and walnuts), and regular consumption of warming broths with immune-supporting herbs and medicinal mushrooms. Get plenty of time outdoors or take a quality vitamin D supplement to support immune function.

PRACTICE: HAVING THE HARD CONVERSATION

When we're under the weather, all sorts of negative feelings can arise. We often want to hide away, feeling helpless, exhausted, feverish, and unworthy. Whether it's coming down with the flu or a herpes outbreak, having a viral infection means we'll need to step up and communicate frankly with loved ones, co-workers, friends, or family members. These conversations don't have to be the end of the world or even a big deal, but they can be scary if you're not used to having them. This can be especially true if it involves a new romantic interest, a friend, or calling into work. Having to admit you need support when you're not feeling well, that you can't make it into work, that you need to reschedule a hangout, or that you must momentarily hit pause on kissing or sex due to an outbreak can bring up a lot of vulnerability. It's perfectly normal to not want to let people down or worry about what someone will think of you, but we can't let these worries and doubts keep us from being honest about where we're at and what we need.

There's a lot of weird stigmas about the common cold, the flu, and especially herpes. You aren't gross, a bad worker or employee, unlovable, dirty, or a burden. Your dating or social life isn't over either. These viruses are incredibly common, and there are many herbal solutions, dietary recommendations, and lifestyle tips that can help with prevention or quicken healing time when sick or having an outbreak. If anything, use this opportunity to create a little network of care between you and your friends. When you're sick, they show up for you, and vice versa, and this way no one feels alone in their time of need.

It's perfectly normal to not want to let people down or worry about what someone will think of you, but we can't let these worries and doubts keep us from being honest about where we're at and what we need.

Here are some sample prompts to guide you in having tough conversations, without apologizing. These can be used as a template for a text message or as inspiration for a phone call or face-to-face chat.

WHEN SICK OR HAVING AN OUTBREAK AND NEEDING SUPPORT:

→ "Hi, I'm super sick, could you bring me some dinner? I'd love some soup or Indian food and can get you back next time you're not feeling well."

→ "Hey, do you have any lemon balm? I'm starting to have an outbreak and I'm out."

→ "Gosh, I'm getting a cold sore for the first time and I'm freaking out. You've always been so upfront about herpes and you know a lot, I wondered if we could meet up and talk? The internet is overwhelming. I'd love some tips or herbal self-care recommendations."

NEEDING TO RESCHEDULE A SOCIAL ENGAGEMENT DUE TO BEING SICK OR HAVING AN OUTBREAK:

→ "Say, I can't make it tonight. I can feel myself getting sick/starting to have an outbreak. I need rest, herbs, and a chill night in. Can we reschedule for a day next week? What day is best for you?"

WHEN NEEDING TO TALK TO A FAIRLY NEW ROMANTIC INTEREST ABOUT HERPES:

→ "Hi there! I'm so excited about our next date in a few days. Work has been nuts this week and I'm starting to get a cold sore. I get them occasionally when I'm stressed and wanted to let you know ahead of time that I have oral herpes. So we should cool it on kissing/oral play until the sore goes away, but there's no reason to not hang out and have fun together in other ways. Let me know if you have questions, there's a lot of misinformation out there. We can touch base via text or when we meet up on Friday."

→ "Hey, I know we're just starting to hang out, but before things get physical, I want you to know that I have HSV-2, genital herpes. It's a pretty common virus that I've lived with for a few years now. I have a bunch of supportive practices set up for myself and being open and honest about it is important to me. Wanna go on a walk in the next few days and talk? I'm happy to answer questions or send some good info your way."

→ "Hi, I'm starting to get sick. I'm going to do everything I can to be okay for my shift (tomorrow, in the next few days, etc.) but I wanted to let you know that I may need someone to cover. Let me know if I can help reach out to people. I'll keep you posted."

→ "Hey, I woke up this morning and feel awful. The flu is going around and I've got it bad. I'm not going to be able to come in today because I'll get others sick and do more harm than good. I don't want to risk pushing myself and staying sick longer or infecting others. Thanks for understanding."

HERBS AND FLOWER ESSENCES

With any viral infection, focus on prevention by supporting your nervous, immune, and lymphatic systems daily with nourishing teas, tinctures, broths, etc. Herbs and foods like ashwagandha, astragalus, gotu kola, holy basil/tulsi, lemon balm, licorice, and medicinal mushrooms (reishi, maitake, shiitake) can strengthen, modulate, and support both the immune and nervous systems, while daily consumption of alfalfa, calendula, cleavers, dandelion, nettle, and red clover can gently cleanse and alkalize the body, moving lymphatic tissue and supporting the liver and kidneys in detoxifying. Viruses thrive on a sugary, acidic diet, so focus on getting plenty of fresh, colorful fruits and veggies and drinking herbal infusions.

At the first sign of symptoms—aches and chills, sores, a runny nose, a scratchy throat, etc.—work with antiviral and immune-stimulating herbs like echinacea, elderberry, ginger, lemon balm, and licorice.

Eat more fresh garlic and cook with onions and aromatic herbs. If you tend to get hit regularly or on a yearly basis with herpes outbreaks or the cold or flu, you should have these herbs and preparations stocked in your home apothecary.

Usually when fighting off any kind of infection, you will want to come at it frequently and hard, hitting it from a range of angles. Take a dropperful or two of tincture every few hours while drinking a strong herbal infusion throughout the day. Having a few different preparations with different herbs gives you more full-spectrum support.

You will also want to include any herbs that target specific issues. For example, if every time you get a cold you get a terrible cough, include angelica, bee balm, elecampane, licorice, oregano, peppermint, or thyme into your routine. Brew a quart jar of a medicinally strong infusion of a combination of these herbs and sip throughout the day, along with drinking plenty of water so you stay hydrated.

Elder (*Sambucus* spp.)

PARTS USED flower, berry

ENERGETICS cooling, drying

Elder is a celebrated medicinal with a rich folk tradition in Europe and North America. Elder varies from a small shrub to a sizable tree, with the berries ripening in late summer and early autumn. Both the berry and flower of elder have traditionally been used in food and medicine, from jams and wines to winter remedies.

Elder flower is a diaphoretic, meaning it induces sweating and moves fevers, working with the body's innate wisdom to heat up and fight infection. Elderberry boosts and balances the immune system and can help reduce inflammation and swelling common in nasal congestion and respiratory complaints.

The berries are a prized remedy for all manner of colds and flu and act as a general immune enhancer. Elderberry inhibits the influenza virus from replicating, making it one of the best allies for flu we have. It's also a great remedy for a sick and fussy child as it is gentle, fast acting, and delicious, and great for an aging family member who needs some broad-spectrum immune support.

WORD TO THE WISE The berries are incredibly delicious when made into syrups or oxymels and gentle enough for all ages, though take special care to always work with dried or cooked elderberries, never fresh. Fresh elderberries contain a compound called *sambunigrin* that can cause vomiting and severe diarrhea if ingested. The flowers do not contain this compound and are safe to work with fresh. If harvesting elderberry from a backyard or the neighborhood, make sure to only pick ripe, darker blue or purple berries.

SUGGESTED PREPARATIONS syrup, decoction, oxymel

FAVORITE PLANT PAIRINGS ginger, elecampane, lemon balm, rose or rose hips

Elderberry–Lemon Balm Oxymel

A yummy alternative to tinctures and syrups, oxymels combine the healing power of honey, apple cider vinegar, and herbs. Use this oxymel during seasonal transitions when you are more prone to germs or allergies or take as a daily tonic to keep herpes outbreaks at bay.

MAKES 8-OUNCE JAR

2 tablespoons lemon balm

2 tablespoons calendula

1 tablespoon dried elderberries

½ inch chopped fresh ginger

½ cup local raw honey

½ cup apple cider vinegar

See page 232 for instructions on making an oxymel.

Enjoy this oxymel to strengthen immunity and digestive fire and to fight viral and bacterial infections. To take, add a few dropperfuls and up to a teaspoon to tea or a glass of sparkling water, or take directly in the mouth. This oxymel is mood-elevating, immune- and lymph-supportive, and a digestive aid.

NOTE: Children under one year old should not be given honey.

Elderberry Chai

The ideal drink for long winter nights, this elderberry chai boosts immunity, fights infection, nourishes respiratory and digestive functions, and improves circulation.

MAKES 4 CUPS

2 tablespoons elderberry

1 tablespoon licorice

1 tablespoon orange peel

2 teaspoons fresh or dried ginger

1 teaspoon pink whole peppercorns

3 crushed cardamom pods

1 cinnamon stick

NOTE: All herbs should be cut and sifted.

See page 223 for instructions on making an herbal decoction.

To make the blend, add all ingredients to a small jar, put the lid on, and shake thoroughly to combine. Label the jar with the blend title, ingredients, and the date you made it. Store the blend out of direct sunlight and it will keep for 8–12 months.

To make Elderberry Chai, you can either infuse the herbs or decoct them. Either way, use 1 heaping tablespoon of the blend for every 8 ounces of water. For a single serving, add 1 tablespoon to a reusable tea strainer or a small pot of water. Alternatively, you can add the blend to a glass jar, French press, or pot and brew up to 32 ounces.

For an infusion, bring water to a boil and pour it over the blend and allow to steep for a minimum of 15 minutes. For a decoction, bring water to a gentle simmer and add the herbs. Cover the pot with a lid and let steep for 5–10 minutes. Turn the heat off and allow to infuse for an additional 5–10 minutes. Drink hot with a little herbal honey and coconut creamer or use this blend to make mulled wine.

Licorice (*Glycyrrhiza glabra*)

PARTS USED root

ENERGETICS moist, slightly warming

Licorice has been used therapeutically in Chinese medicine for thousands of years. Considered an herbal synergist, licorice added to any blend elevates the effect of each herb and assists them in working together to heal the body. For this reason, you will find small amounts of licorice added to most formulas in Traditional Chinese Medicine.

Like marshmallow root, licorice is a demulcent herb, offering cooling, soothing relief to the inflamed mucous membranes of the respiratory system and gastrointestinal tract. It is a top herb for ulcers, sore throat, inflamed sinuses, heartburn, leaky gut, coughs, constipation, and irritable bowel syndrome.

Its genus name, *Glycyrrhiza*, given by first-century Greek physician Dioscorides, comes from *gluko*, "sweet," and *riza*, "root." Its sweet taste can make it a helpful herb for those trying to curb sugar cravings. Licorice is an adaptogen, strengthening the body to better handle stress.

In addition, licorice is an excellent antiviral herb, inhibiting viral replication and stimulating the immune system for those with hepatitis, herpes, flu, and colds. It can be taken internally as a decoction or tincture to fight viral infection and externally as a balm for viral sores such as during a herpes outbreak.

WORD TO THE WISE When taken in large amounts, licorice can increase blood pressure and cause water retention. Taking a high dose is not common, however, as it would require you to ingest over 10 grams, or 10 milliliters (roughly 10 dropperfuls of straight licorice tincture) a day for an extended period of time.

In any case, work with licorice in smaller doses daily so these issues do not arise. Instead of taking licorice alone, try blending with herbs like ginger, marshmallow root, meadowsweet, or nettle, which are diuretic, combating fluid retention while bringing in their own supportive medicine. This can be especially helpful if you tend to have a wet or moist constitution and retain fluid more easily than constitutionally dry types. Remember that a little bit of licorice goes a long way, in both taste and medicinal potency. If you already have high blood pressure or edema, play it safe and work with other herbs.

SUGGESTED PREPARATIONS decoction, tincture, infusion, syrup

FAVORITE PLANT PAIRINGS ginger, elder, lemon balm, nettle, meadowsweet

Daily Viral Support Tincture

This tincture is an excellent preventative remedy for building and strengthening overall immunity while offering extra defense against viral complaints like herpes simplex or flu. This formula will also support and reinforce your nervous system, buffering against stress and overwork.

MAKES 4-OUNCE (120 ML) BOTTLE

40 milliliters reishi alcohol extract
30 milliliters lemon balm alcohol extract
20 milliliters holy basil/tulsi alcohol extract
20 milliliters licorice alcohol extract
10 milliliters cleavers or calendula alcohol extract

See page 235 for instructions on making a tincture.

Take 1–2 dropperfuls twice daily for an extended period—minimum 4–6 weeks—to boost and balance the immune system and prevent viral infections like herpes or flu. This tincture can be added to a few inches of drinking water, added to a smoothie or juice, or put directly in the mouth.

Breathe Easy Tincture

A personal favorite whenever there's even a hint of respiratory woe.
MAKES 2-OUNCE (60 ML) BOTTLE

20 milliliters licorice alcohol extract

10 milliliters sage alcohol extract

10 milliliters thyme alcohol extract

10 milliliters rosemary alcohol extract

10 milliliters cleavers alcohol extract

See page 235 for instructions on making a tincture.

Take 1–2 dropperfuls twice daily for 1–2 weeks if everyone around you is sick or you're recovering and want to continue to protect your respiratory system. In a pinch, for more acute situations, take 2–4 dropperfuls every hour or two at the first sign of getting sick. Whether that's the first signs of a sore throat, a runny nose, sneezing, cough, or sinus tension, this tincture blend should be taken frequently and consistently to halt infection, reduce inflammation, and simultaneously slow the production of mucus in the case of a runny nose or wet cough, while moistening the discomfort of dry sinuses or hot, brittle lungs. This tincture can be added to a few inches of drinking water, added to a smoothie or juice, or put directly in the mouth.

Strong Lemon Balm Infusion for Herpes Outbreaks

A mainstay herbal infusion for anyone with herpes simplex, start drinking a strong lemon balm infusion at the first sign of an outbreak and as support during one.

MAKES 4 CUPS

4–6 tablespoons lemon balm, cut and sifted

To make a strong lemon balm infusion, use 1 heaping tablespoon for every 8 ounces of water. Add lemon balm to a glass jar or French press and brew up to 32 ounces. Bring water to a boil and pour it over the herb, cover with a lid, and allow to steep for a minimum of 15 minutes. Drink hot or refrigerate and enjoy chilled.

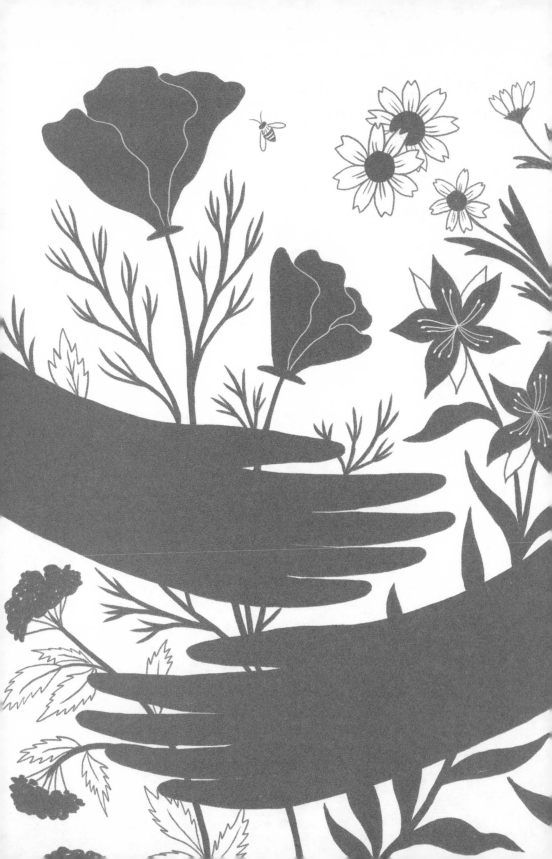

Pain Management

9

LIFE THROWS A LOT AT US, and along the way our body will, at one time or another, experience the physical discomfort (or life-altering effects) of aches and pains. We are strong and resilient. No matter how pain touches your life, from the occasional headache or injury to a more serious relationship with chronic pain, your body isn't broken, and you can find comfort in herbal support, diet, and lifestyle changes.

Pain is a signal, a communication from your body to you. That tension headache, backache, menstrual cramp, nerve pain, reoccurring migraine, joint pain, and so on is letting you know that something you're doing isn't serving your body well. Wow, thanks body! Now that you've gotten the message loud and clear (ouch!), you can empower yourself to make changes that lead to a more comfortable life. Maybe you're needing more rest, less of a certain food or a complete diet overhaul, a change in your work or relationship circumstances, or all of the above. Addressing the underlying cause of your pain will shift or drastically reduce pain.

As you incorporate healthier diet and lifestyle choices, herbs come in to support the vitality of your body by further soothing inflammation, repairing tissues, relaxing tension, and supporting detoxification and circulation.

General Pain and Chronic Conditions

The skeletomuscular and nervous systems are pretty miraculous when challenged and put to the test. The body is constantly working to heal and establish equilibrium. The real trick isn't discovering the one herb to make pain vanish forever; it's learning to listen to your body and not cover up or run from pain. A helpful first step is to ask yourself: *Why is this pain happening?* The answer isn't because your body hates you or because there's something inherently wrong with you. Remember, so much of the work of accepting your body is to get curious and have compassion for yourself. Your body is already trying its hardest to keep you going; all you have to do is figure out how to best support that work.

LIFESTYLE

Lifestyle adjustments depend largely on the kind of pain you have. For chronic conditions, you will want to focus largely on stress reduction, an anti-inflammatory diet (page 66), building a support system and gentle ways to move and care for your body. Managing stress is crucial to dealing with any kind of chronic pain, so take into special consideration how you best relieve stress. Meditation, baths, weekly or monthly check-ins with a therapist or trained herbalist, breathwork, yoga, exercise, walks in nature, fun outings with friends, making art, and journaling are places to start. In addition, bodywork like massage, acupuncture, myofascial release, craniosacral therapy, and chiropractic care can do wonders at loosening tension and adjusting structural imbalances.

In addition, make sure you're getting lots of omega-3 fatty acids, which can be supplemented or found in wild-caught fatty fish like salmon and herring or in walnuts, hemp, flax, and chia seeds. Deficiencies in magnesium and B vitamins are very common in consistently sore, tight, cramping, or twitching muscles, so consider supplementing while seeking out therapeutic foods like oatmeal, quality protein, eggs, brown rice, beans, dark leafy greens, and bone or veggie broth. Seaweed, especially kelp, and nettle are also good sources of magnesium, calcium, and potassium. You can purchase topical magnesium oil to be massaged into sore muscles at most natural grocery stores.

For acute pain—say, an occasional headache, an injury, or sore muscles after a strenuous workout—give yourself time to rest and consider some of the following herbal remedies to help with healing, discomfort, or pain.

PRACTICE: RESTORATIVE YOGA

Unlike most active yoga classes that can have you moving through poses, or asanas, relatively quickly, restorative yoga is a slower-paced, passive, relaxing practice. In this form of yoga practice, you gently move and stretch with the support of props, letting your breath and gravity pull you deeper into a pose. Typically you do fewer poses in a restorative yoga class, holding each for several minutes. This allows you to really slow down, sink into the stretch, and release the busyness of your day, practicing stillness while you breathe and unwind.

Restorative yoga helps calm the nervous system, loosens tension, lessens pain, deepens breathing, and supports restful sleep. It's an excellent way to begin a yoga practice if you haven't practiced yoga before, or if you want to deepen your established yoga practice. You don't have to worry about difficult poses, a hot room, or a fast pace with poses you don't know. Usually the lights are dim and the music promotes tranquility. It's also a great low-impact way to keep your body moving, especially if chronic pain, arthritis, headaches, insomnia, nervousness, anxiety, or depression is an issue. Though it can be practiced at home, seeking out a class offers you a community to engage with, which can uplift your mood if pain tends to keep you isolated and alone.

> Restorative yoga helps calm the nervous system, loosens tension, lessens pain, deepens breathing, and supports restful sleep.

HERBS AND FLOWER ESSENCE

Herbal support for aches and pains comes primarily in the form of muscle-relaxing, pain-reducing, inflammation-soothing, tension-releasing herbs:

- → California poppy
- → Cannabis
- → Chamomile
- → Damiana
- → Feverfew
- → Ginger
- → Kava
- → Linden flower

- → Meadowsweet
- → Passionflower
- → Pedicularis
- → Skullcap
- → St. John's wort
- → Turmeric
- → Valerian
- → Wood betony

Depending on the complaint, severity, and regularity of your pain, your best bet is to work with a few of these herbs in a number of different preparations, ingesting them in infusions and tinctures, taking herbal baths, and applying herbal oils to sore areas on a consistent basis.

If you want to work with flower essences for aches and pains, try star of Bethlehem and/or gentian to start. Star of Bethlehem (*Ornithogalum umbellatum*) helps us restore energy after trauma. Incorporate this if you have been plagued with stress and pain following a traumatic physical event or an emotional shock. Gentian (*Gentianella amarella*) helps when chronic pain flares or a sudden, serious injury has you feeling discouraged and in despair. It can restore our faith in healing, help us to be optimistic, and give us the confidence and certainty to recover.

California Poppy (*Eschscholzia californica*)

PARTS USED whole plant

ENERGETICS cooling

A notable showstopper with its golden blooms, California poppy grows abundantly in the rolling hills and meadows of the western United States and Mexico. It is a botanical ally that offers support for a number of ailments, and it's easy to grow in your backyard. A relative of the infamous opium poppy, California poppy has similar sedative, muscle-relaxing, pain-relieving properties while being a milder, nonaddictive option for pain, insomnia, and mood-related complaints like anxiety and mental exhaustion.

California poppy can be especially beneficial in situations where lack of restful sleep is due to physical discomfort, tension, and pain. If you have chronic pain of any sort, migraines, menstrual cramps, or an injury (especially of the mus-culoskeletal system) that is keeping you up at night, either due to the physical pain or the mental stress, add California poppy to your daily routine and evening sleep ritual. To induce sleep in the evening, pair with passionflower and any other favorite sleep herbs.

California poppy can safely soothe physical and mental agitation simulta-neously. If swirling thoughts, restlessness, nervous jitters, or full-blown anxiety attacks are an issue, whether at night or during the day, this plant can offer you a calming deep breath. Best of all, California poppy is gentle enough for kids, while a higher or more consistent dose can pack a punch for adults. In addition, California poppy can be a formidable remedy for kids if hyperactivity, bedwetting, inconti-nence, toothaches, or colic pains are an issue. In most cases for kids, California poppy pairs wonderfully with chamomile.

WORD TO THE WISE An excellent herbal support to reduce the likelihood of a herpes simplex virus outbreak in those already affected by the virus, California poppy does this by promoting sleep and calming overly stressed-out states, both of which are often triggers for a herpes outbreak.

SUGGESTED PREPARATIONS tincture, infusion

FAVORITE PLANT PAIRINGS passionflower, chamomile, valerian, kava

Tension Tamer Tincture

A useful tincture blend for achy muscles after a strenuous workout or to loosen tension in an overworked body.

MAKES 2-OUNCE (60 ML) BOTTLE

20 milliliters California poppy alcohol extract
20 milliliters meadowsweet alcohol extract
10 milliliters kava alcohol extract
10 milliliters blue vervain alcohol extract

See page 235 for instructions on making a tincture.

Take 1–2 dropperfuls and as many as 3–4 dropperfuls 2–4 times daily depending on severity of tension. This tincture is great when experiencing physical discomfort and aches and pains and will assist in relaxing the body and mind. This blend is ideal for those acute, in-the-moment complaints, like after a long day at work or when you've overexerted yourself. Take some a few times before bed and again, as needed, upon awakening. This tincture can be added to a few inches of drinking water, added to a smoothie or juice, or put directly in the mouth.

Meadowsweet (*Filipendula ulmaria*)

PARTS USED aerial parts

ENERGETICS cooling, drying

Commonly referred to as *queen of the meadow*, meadowsweet is a pleasantly aromatic plant that can be found growing in fields in the eastern United States. Native to Europe and Asia, meadowsweet has a substantial reputation in early European texts and was considered a sacred herb by ancient Druid priests.

Salicylic acid, the chemical precursor for acetylsalicylic acid, or aspirin, has been identified and isolated from meadowsweet leaves. Meadowsweet can thus be consumed for any and all complaints that would warrant the use of aspirin or NSAIDs (nonsteroidal anti-inflammatory drugs, e.g., Advil) without the side effects that include bleeding ulcers and tinnitus. Interestingly, meadowsweet is often used by herbalists to heal the complaints aspirin can create and is an exceptional example of how whole-plant preparations can be more effective and gentler than isolated constituents. Whether for pain, inflammation, or fever, meadowsweet is a potent botanical remedy.

An ally for digestive distress like stomach ulcers, acid reflux, nausea, poor digestion, and leaky gut, meadowsweet heals the tissues of the GI tract while encouraging healthy digestion and reducing pain and inflammation. For GI complaints, combine with calendula, chamomile, ginger, marshmallow root, and/or rose, in addition to making appropriate lifestyle and dietary changes. If headaches or migraines are an issue, work with meadowsweet in combination with California poppy, feverfew, gotu kola, and/or wood betony daily as a tea or tincture. Meadowsweet is cooling while promoting circulation, and is ideal for a hot, pounding headache.

WORD TO THE WISE Taking an herbal bath can be a wonderful way to absorb plant healing benefits and ease pain and discomfort. A bath with meadowsweet can reduce tension, calm nerves, and quiet the mind. Try taking a relaxing, warm bath with Epsom salts and fresh or dried meadowsweet for menstrual cramps, arthritis, headaches, and general aches and pains.

SUGGESTED PREPARATIONS infusion, tincture, bath, oil infusion

FAVORITE PLANT PAIRINGS chamomile, feverfew, blue vervain, wood betony, calendula

Other Herbs for Aches and Pains

Some additional herbs that can offer support, either topically or internally, include:

→ **Arnica** (*Arnica montana*): Applied topically as an herbal oil to sore muscles or a homeopathic preparation to quicken healing time of bruises, aches, and pains. Homeopathic arnica, like the brand Boiron, is helpful with tension headaches, muscle soreness, and quickening the healing time of bruises or after surgery. Arnica is toxic internally and should not be applied to areas with open wounds. Arnica is on United Plant Savers To Watch list, so use responsibly.

→ **Blue vervain** (*Verbena hastata*): A favorite purple-flowered garden herb that will grab you with its bitter taste, blue vervain relaxes tense muscles, aids digestion, calms and settles without being overly sedating and is especially useful for driven type As. This is a great herb if you hold tension in the neck and shoulders or are prone to tension headaches.

→ **Cottonwood bud** (*Populus* spp.): The intoxicatingly sweet fragrance alone is healing, but when the spring buds of cottonwood trees are infused in oil, they transform into a wonderfully pain-relieving remedy for sore muscles. Topical application only.

→ **Crampbark** (*Viburnum opulus*): A beneficial remedy used to relax muscular cramps and spasms as well as painful uterine cramps associated with periods. An infusion, tincture, or massage oil can be used.

→ **Pedicularis** (*Pedicularis* spp.): A favorite herb for muscle tension, stiffness, backaches, general soreness, and pain. Pedicularis is an excellent and safe skeletal muscle relaxant that can be infused in oil, sipped as an infusion, added to baths, taken as a tincture, or smoked in a lovely herbal smoke blend. Unlike kava, pedicularis is not as easy to find commercially, but many species of this tension-soothing plant grow across the country. Find a trusted apothecary or medicine-maker in your region and see if they carry it. Stick to supporting trained herbalists and medicine-makers when seeking out this plant, as it is semiparasitic, meaning that it attaches itself to surrounding host plants and can share the constituents of whatever is growing around it, making it potentially harmful. Therefore you need to be able to not only successfully identify pedicularis but all the plants it is growing near. When I first studied this plant in Oregon, it would commonly grow along patches of poison oak, which would be absolutely terrible to ingest. In addition, depending on where you live, pedicularis may be endangered or at risk.

→ **Peppermint** (*Mentha piperita*): No home apothecary would be complete without peppermint leaf. Infuse in oil for a tingling, muscle-relaxing massage oil, add fresh or dried leaf to a foot soak, sip tea, or massage a few drops of therapeutic-grade essential oil into sore muscles or into your neck and shoulders to soothe a headache.

→ **Willow bark** (*Salix* spp.): Like meadowsweet, willow contains aspirin-like compounds that can offer a mild pain-soothing, inflammation-reducing effect. Tincture or topical application.

Inflammation-Soothing Infusion

Enjoy daily to help combat inflammation, reduce stress, and improve calm.

MAKES 4 CUPS

2 tablespoons meadowsweet

1 tablespoon gotu kola

2 teaspoons rose

2 teaspoons linden flower

1 teaspoon chamomile

NOTE: All herbs should be cut and sifted.

To make the blend, add all ingredients to a small jar, put the lid on, and shake thoroughly to combine. Label the jar with the blend title, ingredients, and date you made it. Store the blend out of direct sunlight and it will keep for 8–12 months.

To prepare, use 1 heaping tablespoon of the blend for every 8 ounces of water. For a single serving, add 1 tablespoon to a reusable tea strainer. Alternatively, you can add the blend to a glass jar or French press and brew up to 32 ounces. Bring water to a boil and pour it over the blend and allow to steep for a minimum of 15 minutes. Drink hot or refrigerate and enjoy chilled.

Headaches

The tricky thing in dealing with headaches is that they are different for each person and vary in their cause and severity. One person may respond to a rosemary foot soak and a cup of chamomile and peppermint tea, while another person may try those and get no relief. The best advice is to start paying attention to your triggers and consider diet and lifestyle changes accordingly. Keep a journal so you can pay close attention to see if your headaches happen around the same time each month; are due to a chronic illness; arise whenever you eat a certain food or are overly stressed; or are due to poor posture, injury, lack of exercise, or dehydration. Recognizing these triggers can help you work with herbs that prevent the pattern or frequency of headaches instead of simply working to treat a headache in the moment. Many of the herbs described in this section work on relaxing tension and fighting inflammation, versus being the kind of powerful painkillers that will numb you, such as over-the-counter or prescription pain relievers.

Stock up on a few herbs that you can consistently work with as daily preventative support: feverfew, holy basil/tulsi, skullcap, and wood betony. In addition, herbs like California poppy, kava, and meadowsweet can be used at the first sign of a headache to bring relief.

LIFESTYLE

Headaches are almost always a symptom of something else, and searching for the root cause can take time. Seek out a trained herbalist or holistic health-care provider to support you. Staying hydrated is huge when it comes to preventing and easing the hurt and duration of any type of headache. Make sure you're drinking on average eight 8-ounce glasses of water a day.

Go on an anti-inflammatory diet (page 66). Do this while taking herbs that support gut healing, soothe inflammation, and strengthen the nervous system to ensure you're healing any broader issues that could be playing into your headaches.

Keep a food journal (page 61) and try to pinpoint more subtle food sensitivities. Sometimes you won't have an immediate reaction to a triggering food, and it may take a day or two for the symptoms of eating that food to arise. For example, if you're keeping a food journal, you're more likely to realize that anytime you eat a lot of dairy or drink too much coffee you get a migraine three days later. Common triggers are caffeine, chocolate, red wine, shellfish, gluten, and dairy, so you can start by eliminating those foods one at a time to see what helps.

Make sure you're getting lots of omega-3 fatty acids from sustainable, wild-caught fatty fish, walnuts, and seeds like hemp, flax, and chia. Deficiencies in magnesium and B vitamins are a very common component of headaches, muscle tension, and pain, so consider supplementing while seeking out therapeutic, nutrient-rich foods like oatmeal, quality protein, eggs, brown rice, beans, dark leafy greens, and bone or veggie broth.

PRACTICE: HERBAL FOOT SOAK

An herbal foot soak is a favorite way to relax the body. If you're the type of person who experiences headaches, tension, mental fatigue, worry, and mental chatter that keeps you from fully relaxing, an herbal foot soak may become one of your favorite new practices. Fresh or dried California poppy, damiana, garden sage, ginger, lavender, meadowsweet, rose petals, or rosemary are some of my favorite herbs to work with.

→ Fill a large pot with water and bring to a gentle simmer.

→ Add herbs of your choice to the pot. If desired, add Epsom salts.

→ Place a lid on the pot and remove from heat. Allow to steep for 10–20 minutes.

→ Either keep the hot water in the pot (if it's large enough to immerse your feet) or pour into a large basin for soaking, whichever you prefer. Add cold water to adjust the temperature, though not too much as you want the water to be as hot as you can stand without burning yourself.

→ Find a cozy place to sit, slowly dip your feet into the water, and relax. Cuddle up with a blanket, sip Joyful Surrender Infusion (page 131), and have a loved one massage your neck and shoulders. Enjoy!

HERBS AND FLOWER ESSENCES

Working with herbs to support you through a headache may require a little trial and error. Start with one or two of the herbs previously mentioned in this chapter for pain and discomfort. A few favorites are California poppy, chamomile, feverfew, skullcap, and wood betony. Blue vervain can be used if you tend to get tension headaches radiating from the neck and shoulders due to overwork and perfectionist tendencies. Another remedy for tension headaches is a topical massage oil or salve. Make your own (page 237) or check out Tiger Balm, a remedy that's been around since the nineteenth century. Composed of 16 percent menthol and 28 percent oil of wintergreen, it can be found at most natural grocery stores and will do the trick in a pinch.

For migraines, your best bet is to develop a relationship with feverfew, a plant that has been researched extensively and used by herbalists not only for migraines but also for other types of headaches as well as inflammation and pain. Feverfew will help alleviate the pain of a migraine, though it's more effective when taken daily for a few months as a preventative. Give this sweet flower a few weeks or months of consistent use to experience the full effects.

If you want to work with flower essences for headaches, try feverfew and dandelion to start. Feverfew is a deeply calming essence that helps release nervous, agitated energy. Feverfew flower essence, tincture, and infusion can be used in combination as a preventative for headaches of all kinds. Dandelion flower essence aids in bringing awareness to longstanding mental and emotional patterns that cause muscle tension, tightness, and pain. This remedy can help you identify the underlying cause of holding tension so you can better release it before it manifests as a tension headache or physical rigidity.

> For migraines, your best bet is to develop a relationship with feverfew, a plant that has been researched extensively and used by herbalists not only for migraines but also for other types of headaches as well as inflammation and pain.

Feverfew (*Tanacetum parthenium*)

PARTS USED aerial parts

ENERGETICS cooling

An easy-to-grow and indispensable herb if you or a loved one suffers from occasional or repetitive headaches, migraines, or pain due to chronic inflammation like arthritis, feverfew eases pain, while long-term use as a tincture or infusion can reduce inflammation. In fact, research shows that feverfew has activity similar to common nonsteroidal anti-inflammatory drugs (NSAIDs) such as aspirin or Advil, without the side effects. Regular consumption of feverfew has been shown to inhibit the synthesis of compounds that promote inflammation.

Feverfew has a long history of use in folk medicine, especially among ancient Greek and early European herbalists. A member of the sunflower, or Asteraceae, family, feverfew is a daisy-like flower that can sometimes be mistaken as chamomile and, in fact, these two pair wonderfully. Simply eating two or three fresh feverfew leaves daily can prevent or ease the severity of migraines. If you don't have access to the fresh plant, an herbal infusion of dried leaves or tincture taken daily can be beneficial as well. If you have digestive issues like nausea, poor appetite, and sluggish digestion, especially in conjunction with migraines or headaches, allow the bitter and aromatic quality of feverfew to improve both.

WORD TO THE WISE If muscular tension and cramping, especially menstrual cramps, are an issue, add feverfew to your herbal apothecary. If PMS symptoms include headaches, anxiety, nervousness, digestive problems, general achiness, or cramping, feverfew can be a true asset in the week leading up to your period (or whenever symptoms show themselves). Feverfew can also help jump-start menstruation if it is delayed. For this reason, check in with your trained herbalist or holistic health-care provider before using feverfew if you are pregnant.

SUGGESTED PREPARATION hot infusion, tincture, herbal bath, or foot soak

FAVORITE PLANT PAIRINGS wood betony, chamomile, California poppy, gotu kola, meadowsweet

Tonic Head Ease Tincture

A combination of wonderfully relaxing, tension-releasing herbs made to be taken daily as a preventative if you have reoccurring tension headaches, migraines, or consistent tension in your neck and shoulders. If stress, mental exhaustion, and the unrelenting drive to "do" play into headaches and tension, this can help with both the headache itself and the mindset that leads to it.

MAKES 4-OUNCE (120 ML) BOTTLE

40 milliliters feverfew alcohol extract

30 milliliters wood betony alcohol extract

20 milliliters gotu kola alcohol extract

10 milliliters blue vervain alcohol extract

10 milliliters milky oat alcohol extract

See page 235 for instructions on making a tincture.

Take 1–2 dropperfuls twice daily for an extended period—minimum 4–6 weeks—to help lessen the frequency and intensity of migraines, tension, and stress. This tincture can be added to a few inches of drinking water, added to a smoothie or juice, or put directly in the mouth.

Tonic Head Relief Infusion

A beloved tea blend for headaches, chronic stress, and tension, especially if poor diet and digestion, lethargy, poor circulation, and nervousness are underlying issues.

MAKES 4 CUPS

2 tablespoons feverfew

1 tablespoon holy basil/tulsi

1 tablespoon gotu kola

2 teaspoons licorice

2 teaspoons rosemary

NOTE: All herbs should be cut and sifted.

To make the blend, add all ingredients to a small jar, put the lid on, and shake thoroughly to combine. Label the jar with the blend title, ingredients, and the date you made it. Store the blend out of direct sunlight and it will keep for 8–12 months.

To make the infusion, use 1 heaping tablespoon of the blend for every 8 ounces of water. For a single serving, add 1 tablespoon to a reusable tea strainer. Alternatively, you can add the blend to a glass jar or French press and brew up to 32 ounces. Bring water to a boil and pour it over the blend and allow to steep for a minimum of 15 minutes. Drink hot or refrigerate and enjoy chilled.

Nerve Pain

Whether it's numbness or the sensation of pins and needles, burning, or pinpricks, nerve pain can disrupt our days and limit our mobility. There are many causes of nerve pain, from bone or joint misalignment causing the nerve to be pinched (as with sciatica), to more complex, chronic conditions like multiple sclerosis and fibromyalgia.

When using herbs and holistic therapies, you want to focus on reducing inflammation, nourishing your nerves, and supporting the overall health of your nervous system.

LIFESTYLE

Altering your lifestyle to address nerve pain depends largely on the cause of nerve pain. If a nerve is being pinched by a joint or bone, prioritize chiropractic care, bodywork like massage or craniosacral therapy, myofascial release, acupuncture, rest, stretching, and bringing awareness to poor posture or activities that could be worsening the issue. Restful sleep, stress management, and exercise are key. Focus on gentle exercises like walking, swimming, and restorative yoga (page 199) if movement is uncomfortable.

If nerve pain is related to more longstanding, chronic issues like fibromyalgia, multiple sclerosis, or diabetes, focus on removing inflammatory foods; recognizing triggering foods; drinking plenty of water; limiting consumption of coffee, alcohol, and sugar; and getting omega-3s and healthy fats. Essential fatty acids soothe inflammation and protect the myelin sheaths that cover nerve axons, which are essential to healthy nerve function. Chronic nerve pain like fibromyalgia can also have roots in past trauma, so see a trauma-informed herbalist and/or therapist or look into a specialist trained in EMDR (eye movement desensitization and reprocessing) for support and relief.

PRACTICE: SELF-MASSAGE
WITH HERBAL OILS

Pausing in your day to massage your body and say thank you for all that it does can be an amazingly grounding self-love ritual. By connecting with the sensations of your body, you gradually encourage calm and embodiment. Daily self-massage also brings greater awareness of how your body looks and feels day to day, which can be helpful for catching a complaint before it becomes serious.

Self-massage can also be a low-cost way to work the areas of your body that are prone to pain, especially nerve-related pain that has an underlying musculoskeletal component. When tight, inflamed muscles or joints swell, break down, or shift out of place, pinching the nerves and causing pain, massaging with inflammation-reducing botanical oils is an excellent practice.

Making your own personal body oils takes self-massage to the next level. Try infusing your choice of oils with some of the following:

→ Calendula   → Meadowsweet

→ Damiana   → Mint

→ Ginger   → Pine

→ Kava   → St. John's wort

→ Lavender   → Violet

The skin is our largest organ of absorption and elimination, so what we put on it—and the intention behind that practice—matters. Carrier oils like almond, apricot kernel, avocado, jojoba, olive, rose hip, sesame, and sunflower offer their own set of moisturizing, antioxidant-rich, healing benefits. These oils diminish dryness and provide essential fatty acids that the body (especially the nerves and nerve endings) depends on. Interestingly, the nervous system relies on healthy fats but to function properly, so not only should we be consuming healthy fats, we can go a step further and use many of those same oils (avocado, coconut, olive, sesame, and sunflower) in our body-care and stress-management regimes.

Depending on your needs, you can make a whole-plant herbal oil as unique as you (see page 237).

HERBS AND FLOWER ESSENCES

Certain herbs are renowned tonics that help rehabilitate, tone, and strengthen the nerves and nervous system. They are known as *neurotrophorestoratives*, herbs with a special affinity for the nervous system. More than other herbs, these plants are well-suited to restoring the vitality of the nerves and building up depleted nervous systems when taken daily for an extended period of time. A few notable herbal neurotrophorestoratives are blue vervain, damiana, lion's mane mushroom, oat (especially milky oat tincture), skullcap, and St. John's wort.

In addition, a mineral-rich, tension-calming, inflammation-reducing, nutritive infusion should be a daily staple. Try making a blend with any combination of

→ Calendula

→ Chamomile

→ Dandelion root

→ Gotu kola

→ Holy basil/tulsi

→ Linden

→ Meadowsweet

→ Nettle

→ Oatstraw

→ Passionflower

→ Rose and/or rose hips

→ Woody betony

Make enough of the blend to keep on hand in a pint or quart jar and consume a medicinal-strength dose (1 cup of infusion, 3 times daily). See chapter 10 (page 219) for more information on preparing and drinking medicinal-strength herbal infusions.

If you want to work with flower essences for nerve pain, try mimulus and cotton grass to start. Mimulus is used when there is a known fear causing anxiety and tension. When we experience pain, especially the debilitating effects of nerve pain, we can find ourselves overcome with fear that the pain will never go away, that we won't get through it. Mimulus calms the fearful voice and gives us the courage to know that healing is possible. Cotton grass aids us in acknowledging the full extent of the core issues that led to an injury or longstanding issue. When you are overly fixated on the complaint instead of the healing process, cotton grass supports you in releasing the physical, mental, and emotional baggage associated with the pain or trauma so you can move forward unencumbered.

St. John's Wort (*Hypericum perforatum*)

PARTS USED flowers

ENERGETICS drying, slightly warming

Blooming around the summer solstice when the days are long and the sun is at its height, St. John's wort is commonly recommended when seasonal or mild depression creeps in and we need a bit of liquid sunshine. In general, long-term use is needed to experience noticeable results. If you tend to get seasonal depression yearly, establish a practice with St. John's wort 4–6 weeks before you usually begin to experience symptoms. If you are interested in getting off antidepressants and looking for herbal options, start a dialogue with your holistic health-care provider or trained herbalist. Remember that lifestyle and dietary changes should also be considered, as depression is a broadly used term with a myriad of root causes.

Overall, St. John's wort is of greater use to those with chronic or nerve-related pain, as it promotes nerve regeneration. Topical St. John's wort is good for sciatica, pinched nerves, or burns, as it restores nerves and reduces inflammation. In addition, this herb is a powerful antiviral and is highly regarded in the treatment of herpes outbreaks when used internally, externally, or both, as well as for shingles or the flu.

WORD TO THE WISE If you are on medication, whether for mood or other complaints, you want to be cautious about working with this plant. St. John's wort has a stimulating effect on the liver that can cause many medications to be metabolized and cleared before they have a chance to work. This is usually why many herbalists do not recommend taking St. John's wort if you are on medication for depression or related complaints.

SUGGESTED PREPARATIONS tincture, body oil, salve

FAVORITE PLANT PAIRINGS milky oat, wood betony, lemon balm, skullcap, calendula

Nerve Nourish Body Oil

A nice complementary treatment for nerve-related pain for everything from sunburn, to shingles, to sciatica.

MAKES 8-OUNCE JAR

> 3 tablespoons fresh St. John's wort
> 1 tablespoon calendula
> 2 teaspoons ginger
> 2 teaspoons peppermint
> 1 cup carrier oil(s) of choice

NOTE: All herbs should be cut and sifted.

See page 235 for instructions on making herbal oil.

To use, massage a quarter-sized amount into hands and massage on clean skin, prioritizing areas that are affected by nerve pain. This oil relieves pain and inflammation.

Some of my favorite carrier oils are organic, cold-pressed, unrefined sesame, olive, almond, and apricot kernel oil. Pick one or combine several.

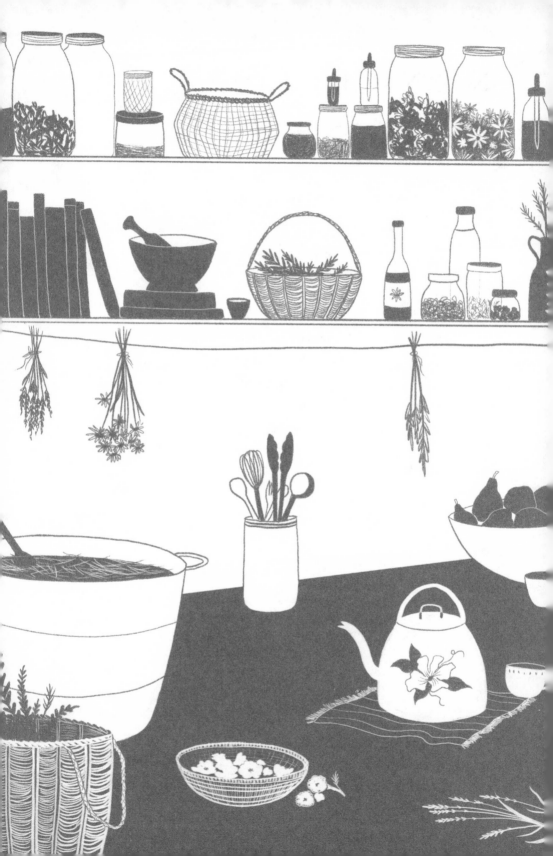

Your Home Apothecary

10

MEDICINE-MAKING RECIPES have been preserved and passed down through the generations. Some herbal preparations have been used and perfected for thousands of years. These traditions were kept sacred and alive by witches and wise women, midwives and medicine men who passed them along from mother to daughter, neighbor to neighbor, teacher to apprentice.

Crafting your own medicines is a form of activism. It is setting an intention—that you, your family, and your community deserve to be well, deserve to have medicines that are both affordable and made from lovingly grown or ethically harvested plants. These medicines are simple and effective, fun to make, and usually quite delicious.

Traditionally, herbs were harvested and medicines made in alignment with the moon, sun, and planets. You may find that this adds greater symbolism to your medicines, but it is not essential.

As a beginner, making medicine can feel bewildering. Don't fret. Once you learn a few basics, you'll find yourself eager to dive in. Always remember to embrace experimentation and play, trust your intuition, and toss out notions of perfection. Though you'll want to keep safety in mind, there is no right way, and with each tincture made and cup of tea shared, you will grow in your craft. Making your own medicine is personal, slow, and creative. You will learn over time what works and what doesn't. The gift of finding your own way is that you will discover which medicines and methods work best for you and yours. You will work with the plants that grow near you, and through this practice build a level of expertise and intimacy with both plant and body.

Crafting your own medicines is a form of activism.

Though there are many different ways to make herbal medicines, in this chapter you will find traditional folk methods for medicine-making. The methods described are intended to be as straightforward and basic as possible. Allow this to be freeing instead of overwhelming. Whether you favor exacting measurements and math equations or your own inner guidance and folk wisdom, there is an approach to medicine-making for everyone, and you are free to use recipes as guidelines to establishing your own creative way.

FOLK METHOD

When it comes to medicine-making, I like to use my intuition and not worry so much about being perfect. I tend to be attracted to self-care practices that bring me into my body and encourage my other information centers—my gut and heart—to guide me. It can be easy to let yourself become overly worried or rigid about following a recipe exactly, especially when you're a beginner. For this reason I prefer teaching a method of preparation called the *folk method* also known as *herbal maceration*, which asks us to rely on our senses. Best of all, this method is straightforward, requires very few tools, and can be used whether we're making an alcohol extract, herbal vinegar, or oxymel.

Basically, you're going to use a clean glass jar with a lid, usually 8 to 12 ounces is ideal for beginners. If you know you want a large batch of something to share, grab a quart jar. No matter the size, fill the jar about three-quarters full with finely chopped herbs, pressing them down to get as much plant matter in the jar as possible. Then cover the herbs with your solvent of choice—alcohol in the case of a tincture, vinegar for an acetum (i.e., herbal vinegar), and vinegar and honey for an oxymel.

There's no measuring, no math, no weighing ingredients: all you need is the jar, plants, desired solvent, and a willingness to trust your senses, experiment, and play.

SIMPLES

Brewing simples is an excellent way to familiarize yourself with plant medicine. Simples are an infusion or tincture using only one herb, which encourages intimacy between person and plant. Try drinking a quart of nettle, lemon balm, or yarrow simple throughout the day for a week or two. Brew it for different lengths of time: 15 minutes, 3 hours, overnight. How does the color, aroma, and taste change?

Take note of how your body responds. There's nothing wrong with buying pre-made formulas at your local health-food store or from a trusted medicine-maker, but if a formula doesn't work for whatever reason, it becomes impossible to tell which plant is the issue. This is why it can be helpful to devote time to getting to know the plants one by one. You may realize you need a sleep formula without valerian, or a digestive formula without chamomile. Remember to pay attention to your body and personalize the process. Once you have gotten to know a plant, you can start blending or formulating in a more intuitive manner.

MEDICINAL-STRENGTH INFUSIONS

Medicinal-strength infusions, whether hot or cold, require a minimum of 10–15 minutes for steeping and at least 1–2 tablespoons of herb per 8 ounces of water.

There is more care and intention when drinking loose-leaf, medicinal-strength infusion that you make yourself. Many herbalists recommend brewing a quart of infusion at a time, since drinking multiple cups of medicinal-strength tea a day is the most effective way to bring your body back into balance. Invest in a French press and use it exclusively for herbal infusions. Keep infusions in a thermos and enjoy them throughout the day, or feel free to reheat or sip cool. You can add honey, herbal syrups, or maple syrup if you like.

If you are seeking to nourish and heal yourself using plants, I encourage you to grow them yourself or find local apothecaries, friendly gardeners, or respected medicine-makers who can supply you with information and herbs. Buy a few ounces of each herb and blend the recipes in this book or come up with your own.

HOT INFUSIONS

This method of brewing is easy and used by anyone who has ever prepared a cup of tea. Aside from simply picking the herbs and eating them, water extractions such as infusions are the ideal solvent to transport the healing properties of an herb from the plant to the body. Hot infusions are usually reserved for the aerial (above ground, flowers and leaves) parts of the plant. All herbs are cut and sifted unless otherwise stated in the recipes in this book.

To begin, find a glass jar, French press, or mug and tea strainer and add 1 tablespoon of dried herbs per 8 ounces of water. Bring the water to a boil and pour over the plant matter, then cover with a lid. Depending on the plants used and taste desired, allow the infusion to steep anywhere from 15 minutes to 8 hours. Medicinal teas are rarely steeped for less than 15 minutes, as it requires some time to fully draw out the healing constituents of the plant. For example, nutritive tea blends with herbs like alfalfa, horsetail, nettle, oatstraw, red clover blossom, and violet leaf are vitamin-rich, so allowing them to steep for eight hours is best. The longer the herbs steep, the more beneficial the brew.

COLD INFUSIONS

Cold infusions are prepared by steeping herbs in cool to room-temperature water. This method is most often used when working with demulcent plants such as marshmallow root. Demulcent plants produce a soothing, cooling, inflammation-reducing mucilage made of polysaccharides (a thick, slimy substance that coats mucous membranes) that high heat will break down. Therefore, this type of extraction is the preferred method when trying to use this aspect of the plant.

To make a cold infusion, use 1 tablespoon of dried herb per 8 ounces of water and steep for up to 8 hours.

Radical Remedies

DECOCTIONS

A different type of water extraction must take place when working with roots, bark, berries, and other less delicate botanicals like reishi. This is due to the tougher, thicker nature of the cell walls, which must be broken down in order to fully extract the medicinal properties. Unlike an infusion, where water is poured over the herbs and allowed to steep for a period of time, a decoction requires that the plant be allowed to gently simmer in a pot of water for a period of time, usually 10 minutes to an hour, although some herbalists recommend even more time in order to retrieve all the restorative goodness. In these cases, a slow cooker would be used. It's important to allow the herbs to simmer on low heat and not boil them, as this would break down the active constituents too much, leaving you with a brew void of vital energy. Always remember that plant medicine is based on a deep respect for the plant as a whole, living organism.

FLOWER ESSENCES

Flower essences are subtle, vibrational remedies for specific emotional states. A flower essence is the energetic imprint of a plant and contains the spirit or intelligence of a plant. By focusing on imbalances in the emotional body, flower essences can bring deep healing and harmony to our mental, emotional, and spiritual selves. Flower essences stimulate our own innate self-healing wisdom and work on a broad range of issues, including depression, creativity, fear, stress, old traumas, and relationships. They are safe for everyone and can be taken internally, added to a bath, or added to other herbal medicine such as a tincture.

Another great thing about flower essences is that they can be made without picking, or harvesting, the plant. This can be a more sustainable model for learning about plants as it allows the plant to continue its life cycle, feed pollinators, go to seed, and maintain the health of the ecosystem it calls home. To make a flower essence without picking the plant, you just need to drape the flower in the bowl of water to the best of your abilities.

Making a flower essence is a time for mindfulness and intention. You may have a specific wish for this medicine or a phrase like *self-love* or *collective healing* in mind that you repeat while making the essence. Dose pattern is typically 4 drops 4 times daily.

Making Flower Essences

An emotional support system you can carry around with you, flower essences are indispensable remedies that are safe for everyone, including pets, the elderly, and kids. Flower essences are a relatively straightforward and hands-off medicine to make at home while encouraging intimacy with the plants and landscape around you. Instead of consuming a generic set of plants that you may have never interacted with, making your own flower essence increases the potency and healing potential.

MAKES 8 OUNCES OF MOTHER ESSENCE

> 8 ounces of spring or filtered water
> Glass or crystal bowl dedicated to essence-making
> Glass jar
> Mesh strainer
> Alcohol, typically brandy
> Labels and a pen

To create an essence at home, you'll need to wait for a sunny, cloudless day or cloudless night if wishing to work with the moon. Find the plant you wish to work with and set up your area, most importantly your glass bowl and spring water. You may wish to create an altar area with candles, photos, or any meaningful object that connects you to the plant and will set the tone for the medicine you'll be making. You're welcome to keep it simple and minimal.

Fill a glass bowl with 8 ounces of water. You don't have to fill the entire bowl.

Either gently drape a flower in the water without cutting it, or cut a few flowers and neatly place in the glass bowl, facing upward. Some herbalists use tweezers or a fallen leaf to pick the plant, others use their hands. If you wish, you can cover the top of the water with flowers, or you can use just one or two flowers. If you have a number that is impactful—say, 4 or 11—you could use that many flowers to make the essence more personal.

There's room for creativity and flexibility in this process, though be mindful of a flower's life cycle and ability to reproduce and the needs of local pollinators in your area. You should never pick all of a flower or plant when working with it and instead only take about 10 percent of what you see.

Allow the essence to sit in the sunlight for at least 1–4 hours, or overnight under the moon. When the essence is finished infusing, preserve it by pouring it through a mesh strainer into a clean glass jar with brandy. A ratio of 40 percent essence to 60 percent brandy will preserve the essence.

You now have a preserved mother essence that you should store in a cool, dark place. The mother essence is not taken directly. To label, mark the plant used, date, and time, plus other meaningful words or an essence name.

To make a stock essence, add 4–10 drops of the mother essence to a 1-ounce (30 ml) bottle filled with equal parts spring water and brandy. You'll want to label this small bottle as well, either with the same information or just the essence title. This can now be carried with you for instant support.

SYRUPS AND ELIXIRS

A syrup is a water-based preparation that is sweetened with local raw honey or raw sugar. Syrups are great for kids, when someone is sick, or to mask the flavor of unpleasant-tasting herbs. An elixir is a syrup with alcohol, usually brandy or vodka, which is added at the very end.

Inspired Combinations

Needing a little inspiration for your next syrup or elixir? Try any of these combinations:

IMMUNE AND RESPIRATORY

→ Elderberry, ginger, cinnamon, yarrow, orange peel (immune boosting)

→ Rosehip, goji berry, star anise, hibiscus (vitamin C boost)

→ Holy basil/tulsi, thyme, mullein, licorice, elecampane, ginger (lung health)

→ Reishi, astragalus, licorice, dandelion root, vanilla bean, cinnamon (immune strengthening)

EVERYDAY NOURISHMENT

→ Nettle, yellowdock root, dandelion root, rose hips, molasses (iron- and mineral-rich tonic)

→ Oatstraw, holy basil/tulsi, lemon balm, damiana (uplifting and nervous system strengthening)

→ Hawthorn berry, reishi, passionflower, motherwort, rosehips (nourishing for heart, immunity, and nervous system)

→ Gotu kola, rosemary, damiana, cacao nibs, holy basil/tulsi (energizing)

RELAXING

→ Kava, passionflower, lavender (chill out, adults only)

→ Chamomile, California poppy, lemon balm, orange peel (chill out, safe for kids)

→ Damiana, hawthorn berry, skullcap, rosehips, cardamom, (promotes grounding and pleasure)

Making Syrups and Elixirs

Adding an herbal syrup and/or elixir to sparkling water, cocktails, oatmeal, or pancakes, or to liven up your cup of tea, is a delicious way to incorporate herbal medicine into your life. My favorite syrups to make are variations on elderberry syrup, though herbal syrup with calming herbs and balancing adaptogens can add extra sweetness and support when times are tough.

MAKES 3 CUPS OF SYRUP OR 4 CUPS OF ELIXIR

1 cup finely chopped dried herbs (see specific recipes)
4 cups filtered water
1 cup local raw honey or sugar, adding more or less to taste
¼ cup brandy (optional for elixir)
Large pot
Mesh strainer or cheesecloth
Jar for storage
Label and pen

To create a syrup, bring the herbs (roots, bark, and/or berries) to a rolling boil in a pot with the filtered water. Immediately from there, partially cover with a lid and turn heat to low so the herbs can gently simmer but not boil. Let this decoction reduce to about half.

Once the decoction has reduced to about half, remove from heat. At this point, you can add any other delicate herbs (leaves, flowers) that don't need to be decocted. Cover the pot with a lid and allow these herbs to steep in the pot for 15–20 minutes.

Next, strain out all the herbs. Once strained, this is your concentrated decoction. Place the strained decoction back on the stove and add the honey or other sweetener of choice. Keep on low heat and stir to help the sweetener incorporate. When using honey, definitely make sure to use low heat, as high heat breaks down the beneficial enzymes. If making an elixir, add the brandy now. Once the sweetener has fully dissolved, let it cool, pour in glass jar or amber bottle(s), and keep in the fridge. Enjoy as you wish!

HERBAL HONEY

Honey is both a food and a medicine, so adding the healing power of herbs only makes for a more potent curative. Honey is the medium by which bees store nectar collected from plants in their hives. Honey has been used as medicine for thousands of years, especially for burns and wound healing, though it can be soothing to inflamed tissue of the upper respiratory system as well. When buying honey for medicinal or culinary benefits, it is crucial that you purchase raw honey. Raw honey is honey that is pure, unheated, unpasteurized, and unprocessed. With a little research and asking around, you may be lucky enough to befriend a local beekeeper and get a direct source. This sweet nectar has antibacterial properties, is a great source of protein and antioxidants, and it contains vitamin C and some B vitamins. When used internally or externally, honey can inhibit the growth of pathogens that are harmful to humans. Honey helps reduce pain and can be used externally on bites, burns, and itches to reduce inflammation. It is also soothing to a sore throat and an ideal ally when someone is getting sick.

Raw honey contains traces of pollen, therefore when local raw honey is consumed regularly it can aid your immune response in not being as triggered to plant pollens in your area, thus helping combat allergies. This only works when consuming local honey from your area. In addition, honey is excellent for the skin and is especially decadent when applied to the face as a mask. It soothes inflammation and moistens dry, irritated skin.

> Honey has been used as medicine for thousands of years, especially for burns and wound healing, though it can be soothing to inflamed tissue of the upper respiratory system as well.

Making Herbal Honey

Making herbal honey is extremely easy. The flavor and color of a particular type of honey will vary based on the types of flower from which the nectar was harvested. Honey has a very complex chemical composition that varies depending on the plant source. The darker the honey, the higher the antioxidant content.

A favorite trick for burns and cuts is to apply a rose petal covered in honey as a bandage. Roses are wound healing, cooling, and anti-inflammatory, and with honey the petals make a soothing germ killer and protective barrier. Stuck with leftover culinary herbs like thyme or rosemary? Try adding these to honey and add to tea next time you're feeling sick. Almost all culinary herbs are antimicrobial and medicinally beneficial.

MAKES 8-OUNCE JAR

3–6 tablespoons Fresh or dried herbs (see specific recipe)
A fine metal strainer (if desired)
Local raw honey

When using fresh herbs, roughly chop, tear, or slightly bruise the herbs. Some recipes may require you to grind the herbs, especially in the case of dried herbs or with roots, berries, and bark. It's recommended to fill the jar halfway if the herbs are fresh and a quarter of the way if the herbs are dry, although adding less of an herb is okay too. Remember, this isn't an exact science. Do what feels right. The more herbs you add, the more you'll be able to taste them in the honey.

Pour the honey on top of the herbs and stir with chopstick or knife to incorporate. Let it sit in a cool, dark spot for at least 7 days, the longer the better.

If you use fresh herbs, say rose petals or lemon balm, you may decide not to strain the honey. After all, the plant matter is edible and a candied treat on its own. However, if you do wish to strain the plant matter, there are a few considerations.

Raw honey can be difficult to strain because it is so viscous. Take a small-to medium-sized pot and fill it with a few inches of water. Add the jar of honey while the water is room temperature and allow the water to slowly warm to a simmer. Occasionally stir the honey, watching as it becomes more liquid. When at the desired consistency, pour the honey through a mesh strainer into a glass measuring cup (for easeful transfer into a jar) or clean, wide-mouth jar with a lid. From there, store in a cool, dark place.

Medicinal Herbs for Pollinators

We owe a lot to pollinators: honeybees and bumble bees, hummingbirds, bats, butterflies, beetles, and all the other animals that support critical ecosystems by helping plants reproduce. Without pollinators, the world as we know it wouldn't function.

All pollinators need a steady supply of nectar and pollen throughout the year, so consider giving back by growing a small plot in your backyard or tending a potted garden on your windowsill or fire escape. Also, think twice before spraying chemicals or uprooting a lawn full of dandelion; many weeds are a medicinal and nutrient-rich food source for humans and animals alike. When planning your garden do some research on the native plants and pollinators in your area and focus on growing those species first and foremost. But here are some medicinally beneficial plants that make for happy pollinators and are easy to grow (or perhaps are already growing in your yard or neighborhood):

→ Alfalfa
→ Bee balm
→ Blue vervain
→ Borage
→ Butterfly weed
→ Calendula
→ Catnip
→ Dandelion
→ Echinacea
→ Fireweed

→ Garden sage
→ Goldenrod
→ Hibiscus
→ Hyssop
→ Impatiens
→ Lavender
→ Lemon balm
→ Lilac
→ Linden tree
→ Milkweed

→ Nasturtium
→ Oregano
→ Peppermint
→ Red clover
→ Rose
→ Rosemary
→ Spearmint
→ Yarrow

HERBAL VINEGARS AND OXYMELS

Herbal vinegars, also known as acetums, are herbal preparations where the herbs are extracted using vinegar, typically apple cider vinegar, which contains potassium and calcium and is mildly antimicrobial.

Vinegar is excreted through the urinary and respiratory systems as well as the skin, so it is most often used to make medicine for the lungs and kidneys and as skin care. Vinegar can be helpful in supporting your body in gentle detoxification and jumpstarting the digestive process, as well as a useful expectorant for respiratory complaints. In addition, vinegars are excellent at extracting minerals and can be used to increase dietary mineral intake. For this reason, working with herbs that are high in minerals (like alfalfa, burdock root, dandelion root, nettle, oatstraw, and rose hips) are a great idea. Consider culinary staples and aromatic herbs like garlic, ginger, holy basil/tulsi, horseradish, lemon balm, onion, rosemary, sage, and thyme as well.

An oxymel is a combination of vinegar, honey, and herbs that has been used since ancient times for a variety of ailments. Oxymels are some of the tastiest preparations in our herbal arsenal, carrying the healing benefits of both honey and apple cider vinegar. This combination makes oxymels especially great at tending to respiratory, digestive, immune, and mood-related issues. Any herb that would be great in herbal honey or herbal vinegar (typically mineral rich, aromatic herbs) is going to be delicious in an oxymel. Other considerations are dried elderberries and/or hawthorn berries and delicately aromatic botanicals like chamomile, elderflower, goldenrod, linden, rose, and violet.

Making Herbal Vinegars and Oxymels

Herbal vinegars can be made and incorporated into any meal. They can be used as mineral-rich, punchy, aromatic salad dressings; added to cooked vegetables or mineral water; or taken in a more medicine-like dose (a few dropperfuls and up to a tablespoon) before meals to help jumpstart digestion. You can use fresh or dried herbs when making herbal vinegar or oxymel.

MAKES 8-OUNCE JAR

> Fresh or dried herb(s) of choice (see specific recipe)
> ½–1 cup organic apple cider vinegar (amount depends
>   on if making herbal vinegar or oxymel)
> ½ cup local raw honey (if making oxymel)
> Fine metal strainer or cheesecloth
> Wax paper
> Label and pen

When using fresh herbs, roughly chop, tear, or slightly bruise the herbs. Fill the jar about two-thirds full with fresh herbs or halfway full with dried herbs. If the herbs are fluffy, you can press them down and add more. If making an herbal vinegar, pour the vinegar over the herbs, filling to the top of the jar and making sure the herbs are completely covered. To protect against corrosion, cover the mouth of the jar with wax paper before applying the lid. Shake to further incorporate the mixture and store in a cool, dark place for at least 7 days and up to 6 weeks.

If making an oxymel, add equal parts honey and vinegar on top of the herbs and stir with chopstick or knife to incorporate. If you know you want your oxymel to be sweeter, add more honey and less vinegar. If you want a tarter, refreshingly sour flavor, add more vinegar and less honey. The great thing about medicine-making is that it's completely customizable, so use this recipe as a jumping-off point for experimentation.

Strain with fine mesh strainer and/or cheesecloth, and make sure to get out as much liquid as possible. Discard the plant material in the compost or trash.

Store the herbal vinegar or oxymel in an amber dropper bottle or glass jar. If kept in the fridge, they can last up to a year; if not, their shelf life is about 6 months.

ALCOHOL EXTRACTS AND TINCTURES

Tinctures are herbal extracts made using alcohol and water as the solvent, or menstruum. Taken orally using a dropper, they are a wonderful and convenient way to take your herbs throughout the day while delivering a potent, fast-acting dose of herbal constituents. The alcohol used in tincturing allows for the extraction of a wide range of medicinally active constituents and is an excellent preservative as well. You can use any spirit you like: vodka is a nice option for beginners as the taste of the herb comes through and it extracts most plant constituents. Brandy is also commonly used as a solvent.

For most plants, an alcohol content of 40 percent to 70 percent is best. To figure out the alcohol content, divide the proof (which is written on the label of whichever alcohol you chose) by two. *Proof* refers to the measure of ethanol (alcohol) in the beverage. For example, the proof of vodka is 100, so the alcohol content in your tincture should be 50 percent, the other half being water. Brandy is 80 proof, therefore the brandy content in your tincture will be 40 percent, the balance of 60 percent being water.

As a rule, the higher the proof, the higher the alcohol content and in turn the stronger the taste of alcohol that will exist in your final tincture. If you've ever taken a tincture and tasted the harsh flavor of alcohol above everything else, it's likely that that tincture was made with grain alcohol. One benefit from higher-proof alcohol is that it gives you a longer shelf life for the tincture.

Making Tinctures

What's nice about tinctures is that they are fast acting, discreet, and easy to carry with you. Tinctures can last a couple of years without degrading the herbal constituents because the alcohol acts as a preservative. Just make sure you keep tinctures in a cool, dark place and preferably store in amber bottles. You can make tinctures with fresh or dried flowers, berries, barks, roots, and leaves.

MAKES 2 CUPS

Herb or herbs of your choice
Pint jar with a lid
Alcohol of your choice—vodka, brandy, or grain alcohol like Everclear
Cheesecloth or mesh strainer
Clean pint jar or amber bottles
Label and pen

Finely chop all the herbs, whether fresh or dried. You can grind the herbs in a spice grinder if you wish. Fill the jar about three-quarters full with herbs. If the herbs are fluffy, you can press them down and add more. Pour the alcohol over the herbs, filling to the top of the jar and making sure the herbs are completely covered. Screw the lid on tightly.

Store your tincture preparation in a cool, dark place. You should shake the jar several times a week; this helps break down the plants cell walls so the constituents are properly extracted, while also sending the medicine good vibes and checking the level of your alcohol. If the alcohol has evaporated so the herbs are not totally submerged, be sure to top off the jar with more alcohol or press down the herbs so they are fully submerged. Allow the tincture to sit for at least 2 weeks, but 6–8 weeks is preferred.

When the tincture is ready to strain, pour through cheesecloth or a mesh strainer into a measuring cup. Make sure to press or squeeze out all the tincture so it doesn't go to waste! The remaining plant matter is known as the *marc* and can be added to your compost bin or thrown away.

Pour the tincture into amber bottles or a freshly cleaned jar. Be sure to label your tincture with its common and/or Latin botanical name along with the alcohol used, alcohol percentage, date made, and anything else that seems relevant.

HERBAL OILS

Infusing herbs in oil creates a versatile ingredient in your home apothecary and kitchen. By infusing dried herbs in oil, called a *carrier oil*, you give yourself the benefit of not only the oil but the herb. Oils typically used as carrier oils have a high concentration of fatty acids, vitamins, and minerals. Combine that with the herbs you're using and your herbal oil has the potential to restore and soften the epidermis and normalize the skin's sebum production, which acts as a protective barrier, locking moisture in and keeping bacteria out, improving skin elasticity, soothing irritation, increasing cell turnover, neutralizing the action of free radicals, and penetrating the skin to deeply nourish and hydrate. And depending on the herbs used (see specific recipes), your herbal oil may also support lymphatic movement and drainage (Lymph Love Massage Oil, page 173), or lessen nerve pain and reduce sensitivity, tenderness, and inflammation (Nerve Nourish Body Oil, page 217).

You're probably already aware that water and oil don't mix. This is exactly why dried herbs are almost always used when making herbal oil. Otherwise, if you were to use fresh herbs, which have water content, you run the risk of the oil going bad due to mold. So if you want to make an oil using fresh herbs that you got from the farmer's market or your garden, let the plants dry out for at least a few days and up to a week before attempting to use them to make herbal oil. There are a few exceptions to this rule, notably when making herbal oil with St. John's wort flowers, as is the case in Nerve Nourish Body Oil. Using the fresh flower is the preferred method for this plant. The outcome is a deep red–hued oil ideal for easing nerve pain and supporting the regeneration of nerve endings.

Making Herbal Oils

Making an herb-infused oil is a wonderfully simple way to incorporate herbs into your favorite skin- and body-care routines. Massage these herbal oils into your skin to help moisturize, reduce inflammation and scarring, encourage circulation and lymph movement, and to relax tense, achy muscles and encourage body awareness and appreciation.

MAKES 8-OUNCE JAR

> Dried herb(s) (see specific recipe)
> 1 cup carrier oil(s) of choice
> Mesh strainer or cheesecloth

To start, finely chop dried herbs or use a spice grinder. Place dried herbs in a clean, dry 8-ounce jar. Generally, you'll fill the jar halfway with herbs, leaving an inch or more of space at the top to cover with oil. Add your carrier oil(s) of choice, give the mixture a stir, and make sure to cover the herbs completely. Herbs should be completely submerged in oil, otherwise they run the risk of attracting mold. Secure the lid tightly and shake well. Keep the jar in a warm, dry spot—by a window or above the fridge, for example—and allow to steep for 3–6 weeks, shaking occasionally. If a few pieces of plant material do float to the top of the oil that is generally okay, but keep an eye out for mold. If any mold forms, immediately spoon off the top layer.

After 3–6 weeks, strain the herbs using a cheesecloth or mesh strainer. Make sure to squeeze out as much oil as possible.

Store in a jar or in amber bottles and use as a massage, face, or body oil; or turn it into salves, lip balms, creams, or as a culinary oil. Store the oil in a dry spot out of direct sunlight and it will last up to 12 months. Carrier oils like jojoba, olive, coconut, or vitamin E oil can be added to increase the shelf life of your oil blend. Always check the smell and look of your oil for signs that it has gone rancid or has mold growing on the top.

Some of my favorite carrier oils for skin and body care are organic, cold-pressed, unrefined almond, apricot kernel, argan, borage seed, coconut, jojoba, olive, rose hip, sea buckthorn, and sunflower. Pick one or combine several. When making herbal oil for culinary uses, stick with carrier oils that you typically cook with like coconut, olive, sesame, and/or sunflower.

ESSENTIAL OILS, HYDROSOLS, AND SUSTAINABILITY

Essential oils, hydrosols (also known as botanical water), and aromatherapy are becoming increasingly popular. Aromatherapy uses our sense of smell to help us relax, feel more grounded, combat depression, uplift mood, and provide a sense of safety. You can access this form of medicine anytime you use your sense of smell to inhale healing plant aromatics—smelling a flower in the park, spraying yourself with hydrosol, and anointing yourself with a fragrant perfume.

Many people are confused about what exactly essential oils are and how they should be safely and correctly used. Essential oils are extremely concentrated plant oils that have been extracted from the plant through a number of processes, most commonly using a distillation still. Note that essential oils and herb-infused oils are different. During the distillation process, the plant's volatile oils are separated from the water-soluble compounds and remaining plant material and collected. To make your own essential oil is pretty advanced medicine-making and requires you to purchase, or know someone with, a still.

Hydrosols are made using a still as is used when making essential oils, but unlike essential oils, hydrosols are a much more sustainable and gentle option when working with plant aromatics. There's a lot of amazingly healing nutrients and plant acids in botanical waters that balance and restore the skin's natural pH. Hydrosols like rose water have been used in culinary traditions and in the skin-care industry for quite a while. They are gentle and safe for all ages. These botanical waters can be used whenever you would reach for essential oils or benefit from plant aromatics, like when you're feeling anxious, ungrounded, restless, overwhelmed, depressed, or agitated, or when dealing with skin distress like acne, inflammation, dry skin, etc. Not only are hydrosols effective for mind, body, and spirit but they also don't require as much plant material to make, meaning their production is more earth friendly and therefore a much better alternative to essential oils from the standpoint of sustainability. Using the same amount of plant material you may get a gallon of hydrosol and only a few drops of essential oil.

It can be tempting to purchase inexpensive essential oils, but buying quality, organic, therapeutic-grade essential oils really do make a difference. Oftentimes, inexpensive essential oils are made with plants that have been sprayed with chemical herbicides and can include fillers that aren't good for humans. Furthermore, it takes about sixty roses to make just one drop of rose essential oil. Think about all the resources it took to create that medicine and how important it is that these plants are grown mindfully, with sustainable practices at the forefront. Hydrosols,

Radical Remedies

however, are less cost prohibitive because they don't require as much plant material; they are usually sold in 2- or 4-ounce bottles, meaning you get a lot more than the typical bottle of essential oil.

Essential oils are almost always used for external use and should be put in carrier oils like almond, coconut, jojoba, olive, etc., or added to an aromatherapy diffuser and inhaled through the lungs. Because the skin is the largest organ of absorption, adding a few drops of essential oils to a body oil, scrub, or bath is the preferred method of application. That said, *please do not add essential oils to any beverage or food and consume them*. Essential oils are powerfully concentrated, volatile aroma compounds and have the potential to damage your liver and mucous membranes and generally irritate your body. If you want to flavor your water, add a splash of hydrosol, or use fresh fruits, cucumbers, or steeped herbs like peppermint soaked in cold water overnight.

Resources

WEBSITES

American Botanical Council: abc.herbalgram.org

American Herbalists Guild: www.americanherbalistsguild.com

Jim McDonald's Master Herbal Article Index: herbcraft.org/articleindex.html

Learning Herbs: learningherbs.com

Sustainable Herbs Program: sustainableherbsproject.com

United Plant Savers: unitedplantsavers.org

BOOKS AND ZINES

HERBALISM

Christine Buckley, *Plant Magic: Herbalism in Real Life*

Rosalee de la Forêt and Emily Han, *Wild Remedies: How to Forage Healing Foods and Craft Your Own Herbal Medicine*

Rosemary Gladstar, *Herbs for Stress & Anxiety: How to Make and Use Herbal Remedies to Strengthen the Nervous System*

Rosemary Gladstar, *Rosemary Gladstar's Medicinal Herbs: A Beginner's Guide: 33 Healing Herbs to Know, Grow, and Use*

Maria Noël Groves, *Body into Balance: An Herbal Guide to Holistic Self-Care*

David Hoffmann, *Medical Herbalism: The Science and Practice of Herbal Medicine*

Janet Kent, *Ease Your Mind: Herbs for Mental Health*

Janet Kent, *Under Pressure: Herbs for Resilience*

Kathi Keville and Mindy Green, *Aromatherapy: A Complete Guide to The Healing Art*

Michele Elizabeth Lee, *Working the Roots: Over 400 Years of Traditional African American Healing*

Phyllis D. Light, *Southern Folk Medicine: Healing Traditions from the Appalachian Fields and Forests*

David Winston and Steven Maimes, *Adaptogens: Herbs for Strength, Stamina, and Stress Relief*

Matthew Wood, *The Earthwise Herbal, Volume I: A Complete Guide to Old World Medicinal Plants*

Matthew Wood, *The Earthwise Herbal, Volume II: A Complete Guide to New World Medicinal Plants*

ELEMENTAL HERBALISM AND HERBAL ENERGETICS

Rosalee de la Forêt, *Alchemy of Herbs: Transform Everyday Ingredients into Foods and Remedies That Heal*

Sajah Popham, *Evolutionary Herbalism: Science, Spirituality, and Medicine from the Heart of Nature*

Michael Tierra, *Planetary Herbology*

Matthew Wood, *The Practice of Traditional Western Herbalism: Basic Doctrine, Energetics, and Classification*

FLOWER ESSENCES

Patricia Kaminski and Richard Katz, *Flower Essence Repertory: A Comprehensive Guide to North American and English Flower Essences for Emotional and Spiritual Well-Being*

MEDICINE-MAKING

Thomas Easley and Steven Horne, *The Modern Herbal Dispensatory: A Medicine-Making Guide*

Rosemary Gladstar, *Rosemary Gladstar's Herbal Recipes for Vibrant Health: 175 Teas, Tonics, Oils, Salves, Tinctures, and Other Natural Remedies for the Entire Family*

James Green, *The Herbal Medicine-Maker's Handbook: A Home Manual*

Sharol Marie Tilgner, *Herbal Medicine from the Heart of the Earth*

PLANT IDENTIFICATION AND REGIONAL FIELD GUIDES

Thomas J. Elpel, *Botany in a Day: The Patterns Method of Plant Identification*

Michael Moore, *Medicinal Plants of the Desert and Canyon West*

Michael Moore, *Medicinal Plants of the Mountain West*

Michael Moore, *Medicinal Plants of the Pacific West*

NUTRITION AND COOKBOOKS

Sarah Kate Benjamin and Summer Singletary, *Be Radical, Eat Traditional! Cookbook*

Sarah Kate Benjamin and Summer Singletary, *The Kosmic Kitchen Cookbook: Everyday Herbalism and Recipes for Radical Wellness*

Amy Chaplin, *Whole Food Cooking Every Day: Transform the Way You Eat with 250 Vegetarian Recipes Free of Gluten, Dairy, and Refined Sugar*

Marc David, *Nourishing Wisdom: A Mind-Body Approach to Nutrition and Well-Being*

Aran Goyoaga, *Cannelle et Vanille: Nourishing, Gluten-Free Recipes for Every Meal and Mood*

Heidi Swanson, *Super Natural Every Day: Well-Loved Recipes from My Natural Foods Kitchen*

FERMENTATION

Sandor Ellix Katz, *The Art of Fermentation: An In-Depth Exploration of Essential Concepts and Processes from around the World*

René Redzepi and David Zilber, *The Noma Guide to Fermentation: Including Koji, Kombuchas, Shoyus, Misos, Vinegars, Garums, Lacto-Ferments, and Black Fruits and Vegetables*

OTHER

adrienne maree brown, *Emergent Strategy: Shaping Change, Changing Worlds*

adrienne maree brown, *Pleasure Activism: The Politics of Feeling Good*

Marlee Grace, *How to Not Always Be Working: A Toolkit for Creativity and Radical Self-Care*

Marlee Grace, *How a Photo and Video-Sharing Social Networking Service Gave Me My Best Friends, True Love, a Beautiful Career, and Made Me Want to Die*

Robin Wall Kimmerer, *Braiding Sweetgrass: Indigenous Wisdom, Scientific Knowledge, and the Teachings of Plants*

Resmaa Menakem, *My Grandmother's Hands: Racialized Trauma and the Pathway to Mending Our Hearts and Bodies*

Jennifer Nelson, *More Than Medicine: A History of the Feminist Women's Health Movement*

Jenny Odell, *How to Do Nothing: Resisting the Attention Economy*

Jennifer Patterson, *The Power of Breathwork: Simple Practices to Promote Wellbeing*

Catherine Price, *How to Break Up with Your Phone*

Bessel van der Kolk, *The Body Keeps the Score: Brain, Mind, and Body in the Healing of Trauma*

Jennifer Williams, *The Actual Feeling: Discussion Questions to Name Emotions and Ask for the Support You Need*

WHERE-TO-BUY GUIDE

Now that you're excited about bringing herbs into your self-care routine, you're probably wondering where to find them. In the long term, it can be extremely empowering to grow your own herbs and have your favorite plant allies growing in your own backyard. I can't recommend this enough!

In the meantime, purchase bulk herbs from small-scale herb growers and support medicine-makers in your community, state, and region as often as possible. Included in this book is a list of growers, herbalists, and suppliers, but this is in no way exhaustive, and I urge you to do some research. Many local farms grow medicinal herbs but don't believe there is a true demand for these plants. Let's change that. Seeking out local and regional medicine-makers or apothecaries is an excellent way to engage with herbalists as well. Many have information-rich blogs, teach classes, offer seasonal CSH (community-supported herbalism) shares, and have social media where they share their passion for plant medicine and healing.

BULK HERBS

Black Locust Gardens, Michigan: blacklocustgardens.com

Cutting Root Apothecary and Farm, Pennsylvania: cuttingroot.com

Fox Trot Herb Farm, Massachusetts: foxtrotherbfarm.com

Freedom Food Farm, Massachusetts: freedomfoodfarm.com

Friends of the Trees Society, Pacific Northwest: friendsofthetrees.net

Frontier Herbs, Iowa: frontiercoop.com

Gentle Harmony Farm, North Carolina: gentleharmonyfarm.com

Healing Spirits Herb Farm, New York: healingspiritsherbfarm.com

Herban Ayurveda, Minnesota: herbanayurveda.com

Mountain Rose Herbs, Pacific Northwest: mountainroseherbs.com

Oshala Farm, Oregon: oshalafarm.com

Pacific Botanicals, Oregon: pacificbotanicals.com

Sawmill Herb Farm, Massachusetts: sawmillherbfarm.com

Steadfast Herbs, California: steadfastherbs.com

Zack Woods Farm, Vermont: zackwoodsherbs.com

MUSHROOMS

Forest Folk Fungi, Tennessee: forestfolkfungi.com

Mycopolitan Mushroom Company, Pennsylvania: mycopolitan.com

MycoSymbiotics, Pennsylvania: mycosymbiotics.net

North Spore, Maine: northspore.com

Smugtown Mushrooms, New York: smugtownmushrooms.com

SEAWEED

Atlantic Holdfast, Maine: atlanticholdfast.com

Island Herbs, Washington: ryandrum.com

Maine Seaweed LLC, Maine: theseaweedman.com

FLOWER ESSENCES

Alaskan Essences, Alaska: alaskanessences.com

Desert Alchemy Flower Essences, Arizona: desert-alchemy.com

Flower Essence Services, California: store.fesflowers.com

Santa Barbara Quantum Health, California: sbquantumhealth.com

Sister Spinster, New York: sisterspinster.net

Sophia Rose, Texas: www.laabejaherbs.com

Sun Song, California: shop-sunsong.com

MEDICINE-MAKING SUPPLIES, TINS, BOSTON ROUND BOTTLES, ETC.

Berlin Packaging: berlinpackaging.com

TRUSTED MEDICINE-MAKERS

69 Herbs, New York

Avena Botanicals, Maine

Corpus Ritual, New York

Dori Midnight, Massachusetts

Fat of the Land, New York

Good Fight Herb Co., New York

Herban Cura, New York

Jam Haw Herbals, California

La Luneria, California

Maypop Community Herb Shop, New Orleans

Ms. Tea Botanica, California

Moon Mother Apothecary, New York

Rebecca's Herbal Apothecary and Supply, Colorado

Ritual Botanica, North Carolina

Rootwork Herbals, New York

Sacred Vibes Apothecary, New York

Snakeroot Apothecary, California

Sundial Medicinals, Utah

Suntrap Botanical, New York

Tucson Herb Store, Arizona

Urban Moonshine, Vermont

Wooden Spoon Herbs, Georgia

Zizia Botanicals, California

Indexes

HERBS AND PLANTS

coffee, 34, 37, 66, 213; replacements for, 24, 52, 82, 83, 87, 105, 109

comfrey, 16

cotton grass, 27, 215

cottonwood bud, 204

crampbark, 204

D

damiana, 21, 23, 25, 26, 30, 159; for anxiety, 110, 117; Banish the Blues Tincture, 161; for brain function, 89; for digestion, 50, 63; Enliven Elixir, 160; Grounded Infusion, 117; for mood, 38, 155, 160, 161, 226; for pain, 200, 208, 214, 215; pairings with, 90, 103, 112, 116, 156, 226; Sacred Spark Infusion, 87; for sleep, 134; for stress, 102

dandelion, 16, 24, 25, 26, 27, 30, 51, 230; Ashwagandha Golden Milk, 85; for digestion, 50–52, 64, 179, 188; for headaches, 209; for immunity, 171, 179, 226; for nervous system, 215; nutrients in, 78, 100, 231; Roasted Dandelion Coffee Replacement, 24, 52; for stress, 102; Trust Your Gut Infusion, 64

devil's claw, 27, 62

E

echinacea, 21, 171, 177, 188, 230

elder, 16, 21, 25, 26, 30, 189; chai, 23, 24, 191; for immunity, 167, 177, 182, 188; Lemon Balm Oxymel, 190; pairings with, 57, 150, 156, 179, 192; preparations of, 226, 227, 231

elecampane, 21, 21, 23, 24, 26, 31, 179; for digestion, 56; pairings with, 57, 189; Release Grief Tincture, 152; Respiratory Aid Tincture, 181; for respiratory health, 69, 177, 181, 182, 188, 226; Thyme Honey, 24, 180

eleuthero, 155

evergreens, 16, 175, 182. See also pine

F

fennel, 21, 51, 62, 63, 64, 129; Trust Your Gut Infusion, 64

feverfew, 16, 25, 26, 27, 50, 203, 210; for pain, 200, 207, 209; Tonic Head Ease Tincture, 211; Tonic Head Relief Infusion, 212

fireweed, 230

flax seeds, 100, 186, 198, 208

flower essences, 27, 223–25; for depression, 155; for difficult emotions, 146, 148; for digestion, 62; for gut healing, 68; for headaches, 209; for mental clarity, 89; for nervous system, 215; in other preparations, 52, 128, 148, 152, 157, 160, 161; for pain, 200;

for relaxation, 125; for sleep, 134; for stress, 102; for vitality, 81

frankincense, 175

fungi, 5, 8, 25, 67, 164, 167, 182, 215. See also reishi

G

garlic, 21, 23, 31, 51, 89, 155, 231; digestion and, 56, 59; immunity and, 165, 167, 177, 178, 182, 188

gentian, 50, 52, 200

ginger, 25, 26, 57, 231; Brain-Boosting Infusion, 95; for brain function, 89, 95; for digestion, 57–58, 62, 67, 203; Elderberry Chai, 191; Elderberry–Lemon Balm Oxymel, 190; Elecampane and Thyme Honey, 180; Ginger Lemon Infusion, 58; Immune Upkeep Tincture, 169; for immunity, 165, 167, 169, 177, 178, 182, 188, 226; Lemon Balm and Orange Peel Honey, 158; for mood, 38, 155, 159; Nerve Nourish Body Oil, 217; for pain, 200, 208; pairings with, 72, 90, 150, 156, 168, 179, 189, 192; preparations of, 214, 217, 231; Sacred Spark Infusion, 87; as warming, 19, 21, 21, 22, 23, 30, 31

ginkgo, 89, 93; Brain Tonic Tincture, 92

ginseng, 37, 78, 79, 155

goji berries, 24, 67, 226

goldenrod, 16, 177, 230, 231

gotu kola, 21, 24, 25, 30, 93, 188; for brain function, 89, 91, 92, 95; Brain Tonic Tincture, 92; Brain-Boosting Infusion, 95; Grounded Focus Tincture, 91; Gut-Healing Infusion, 73; for headaches, 203, 211, 212; Inflammation-Soothing Infusion, 206; for nerve pain, 215; pairings with, 57, 90, 210; for relaxation, 125; Rose Facial Oil, 24, 94; Tonic Head Ease Tincture, 211; Tonic Head Relief Infusion, 212; Trust Your Gut Infusion, 64; Uplift Infusion, 157; for vitality, 78, 79, 226

greens, 23, 24, 30, 34, 49, 50, 67, 186; minerals in, 100, 198, 208

H

hawthorn, 16, 21, 23, 25, 26, 29, 31, 147; for anxiety, 110, 115, 117, 118; Be Cool Iced Tea, 115; for boundaries, 36, 128; Enliven Elixir, 160; Grounded Infusion, 117; Hawthorn Rose Honey, 23, 148, 149; Heart Renewal Tincture, 148; Joyful Surrender Infusion, 131; Joy of Missing Out Tincture, 128; for mood, 146, 148, 155, 160; pairings with, 114, 150, 159, 179, 226; for stress, 102; Sweet Acceptance Tincture, 118

nori, 21, 24, 100

nutritives, 25, 75–77, 78, 81, 134, 226. *See also specific herbs*

nuts, 24, 34, 49, 66, 67, 133, 165, 184 186

O

oak, 27, 81, Joy of Missing Out Tincture, 128

oats, 21, 24, 25, 30, 103, 111, 155, 215; baths with, 24, 69; for brain function, 89, 91, 92; Brain Tonic Tincture, 92; Grounded Focus Tincture, 91; Honey Mallow Soothing Face Mask, 71; Milky Oat, Ashwagandha, and Rose Tincture, 24, 104; as nutritive, 78, 81, 100; pairings with, 82, 84, 86, 126, 216; preparations of, 222, 226, 231; for relaxation, 125, 127; Release Grief Tincture, 152; Restful Slumber Tincture, 138; Skullcap Bedtime Infusion, 139; for sleep, 127, 134, 138; for stress, 102, 105, 106; Stress Less Infusion, 105; Tonic Head Ease Tincture, 211; Trust Your Ease Syrup, 106

olive oil, 24, 34, 155, 237

onions, 31, 56, 59, 67, 179, 231; immunity and, 165, 167, 177, 178, 188

orange peel, 179, 226; Elderberry Chai, 191; Elecampane and Thyme Honey, 180; Lemon Balm Honey, 158; Trust Your Ease Syrup, 106

oregano, 165, 175, 178, 183, 188, 230

Oregon grape root, 183

P

palo santo, 176

passionflower, 21, 23, 25, 26, 31, 103, 137; for anxiety, 22, 29, 107, 110, 111, 113; Don't Panic! Acute Tincture, 113; Joyful Surrender Infusion, 131; Lights-Out Sleep Tincture, 136; for pain, 200, 215; pairings with, 84, 112, 114, 126, 134, 135, 201, 226; for relaxation, 125, 131, 139; Restful Slumber Tincture, 138; for sleep, 127, 133, 134, 136, 138; Skullcap Bedtime Infusion, 139; Sustained Calm Infusion, 139

pennywort. *See* gotu kola

pepper, 89, 155, 165; Elderberry Chai, 191

peppermint, 16, 62, 89, 205, 230; Be Cool Iced Tea, 115; for immunity, 167, 175, 182, 188; Nerve Nourish Body Oil, 217

pine, 16, 21, 24, 41, 175, 182, 214

plantain, 16, 21, 65, 68, 69

poppy. *See* California poppy

R

red clover, 21, 78, 188, 222, 230

red root, 171, 172, 177

reishi, 8, 21, 25, 30, 31, 168, 223; broth, 167; Daily Viral Support Tincture, 193; Immune Upkeep Tincture, 169; for immunity, 164, 167, 169, 177, 188; Joy of Missing Out Tincture, 128; for mood, 38, 155; pairings with, 93, 226; for relaxation, 102, 125, 128; Release Grief Tincture, 152

rose, 17, 21, 21, 23, 25, 26, 31, 150, 230; for anxiety, 111, 115; Be Cool Iced Tea, 115; carrier oil, 237; for digestion, 203; Enliven Elixir, 160; essential oil, 238; Gotu Kola Rose Facial Oil, 94; Gut-Healing Infusion, 73; Hawthorn Rose Honey, 149; Honey Mallow Soothing Face Mask, 71; Inflammation-Soothing Infusion, 206; Joyful Surrender Infusion, 131; Milky Oat, Ashwagandha, and Rose Tincture, 24, 104; for mood, 38, 129, 146, 149, 155, 179; nutrients in, 78, 226; for pain, 208, 214, 215; pairings with, 69, 72, 86, 112, 114, 116, 156, 159, 168, 189, 203; preparations of, 231, 237, 238; for relaxation, 125, 131, 134, 139; Release Grief Tincture, 152; for skin, 69; for stress, 102, 106; Sustained Calm Infusion, 139; Trust Your Ease Syrup, 106; water, 23, 150, 238; wild, 27, 62; for wounds, 229

rosemary, 17, 21, 23, 25, 26, 30, 90, 230; for anxiety, 110; as aromatic, 62, 89; Banish the Blues Tincture, 161; Brain Tonic Tincture, 92; Breathe Easy Tincture, 194; for depression, 155, 161; Grounded Focus Tincture, 91; for immunity, 165, 175, 177, 178, 183, 229; for pain, 208; pairings with, 93, 159, 226; preparations of, 24, 41, 175, 231; Respiratory Aid Tincture, 181; Sacred Spark Infusion, 87; Tonic Head Relief Infusion, 212

S

sage, 16, 21, 50, 110, 208, 230, 231; as aromatic, 62, 89; Breathe Easy Tincture, 194; burning of, 24, 41, 175; for immunity, 175, 177, 178, 183; white, 176

St. John's wort, 25, 26, 30, 155, 216, 236; Nerve Nourish Body Oil, 217; for pain, 200, 214, 215; pairings with, 116, 156

sauerkraut, 23, 54–55, 165

schisandra, 78

seaweeds, 21, 24, 30, 56, 100, 198

self-heal, 27, 102

shiitakes, 67, 164, 167, 168, 188

skullcap, 21, 23, 25, 26, 31, 126; for addiction, 103; for anxiety, 22, 29, 111; for brain function, 89; for depression, 155; for headaches, 207, 209; Joy of Missing Out Tincture, 128;

AILMENTS OR AREAS OF CONCERN

Roasted Dandelion Coffee Replacement, 52; *See also* detoxification

lungs, 31, 174–81, 183; Breathe Easy Tincture, 194; herbs for, 177, 178, 226; practices to support, 109, 175; preparations for, 231, 238–39; Respiratory Aid Tincture, 181

lymphatic system, 30, 170–73; Lymph Love Massage Oil, 24, 173

M

memory, 46, 59, 75, 88–89, 99, 121; herbs for, 79, 89, 90, 93, 103

menstruation, 51, 61, 107, 170, 197; herbs for cramps, 57, 82, 103, 129, 201, 203, 204, 210; herbs to induce, 57, 114

mental clarity, 75–79, 88–95, 208; Brain-Boosting Infusion, 95; Brain Tonic Tincture, 92; Grounded Focus Tincture, 91; herbs for, 76–79, 89–90, 93, 159, 168; phone use and, 88–89; stress and, 102, 105; Stress Less Infusion, 105; Tonic Head Ease Tincture, 211

motion sickness, 57

mucous membranes, 69, 163, 164, 192, 222, 239

mucus, 21, 174, 177, 179, 194

multiple sclerosis, 213–17

muscles, 10, 34, 47, 170, 214, 237; cramps in, 82, 103, 114, 198; soreness in, 199, 204, 205; tension in, 112, 129, 156, 200, 201, 203, 209, 210; Tension Tamer Tincture, 202

N

nausea, 57, 203, 210

nervous system, 29, 30, 79, 122, 226; anxiety and, 107, 111; Daily Viral Support Tincture, 193; diet and, 100, 165, 167; digestive system and, 59, 60, 159; enteric, 45–46, 116; Grounded Focus Tincture, 91; herbs to calm, 22, 29, 63, 103, 111–12, 114, 135, 137, 168, 203; herbs to strengthen, 62, 82, 84, 89, 90, 93, 126, 134, 155, 159, 214–16, 226; immune system and, 166, 184, 188; Nerve Nourish Body Oil, 24, 217, 236; pain, 137, 197, 213–17, 236; Roasted Dandelion Coffee Replacement, 52; self-care for, 124, 132, 199, 213, 214; sleep and, 134; stress and, 59, 100, 103; Stress Less Infusion, 105; Sustained Calm Infusion, 139

P

pain, 21, 126, 228; diet and, 76, 198, 207–8, 213; from headaches, 207–12; herbs for, 57, 159, 168, 200–1, 203–5; Inflammation-Soothing Infusion, 206; Nerve Nourish Body Oil, 217; from nerves, 213–17; practices to counter, 198–99, 207–8, 213–14; Tension Tamer Tincture, 202; Tonic Head Ease Tincture, 211; Tonic Head Relief Infusion, 212

panic attacks, 26, 109, 111; Don't Panic! Acute Tincture, 113

pedicularis, 200, 205

pleasure. *See* joy

pregnancy, 57, 114, 210

productivity, 1, 37, 42, 84, 97–98, 119, 121

professional help, 10, 35, 101, 107, 132, 207; from bodyworkers, 101, 145, 153, 198, 213; from herbalists, 12–13, 35, 101, 103, 107, 111, 155, 205; from therapists, 35, 41, 101, 144–45, 153, 154

R

relaxation, 23, 37, 121–31, 153; herbs for, 125–26, 129, 137, 226; immunity and, 185–88; Joyful Surrender Infusion, 131; Joy of Missing Out Tincture, 128; regenerative practices for, 122–25; Sustained Calm Infusion, 139; *See also* fatigue; sleep

respiratory system, 20, 21, 22, 165, 174–81; Breathe Easy Tincture, 194; Elderberry Chai, 191; Elecampane and Thyme Honey, 180; herbs for, 69, 90, 177–79, 189, 192, 216; preparations for, 90, 175–76, 226, 228, 231, 239; Respiratory Aid Tincture, 181; *See also* viral infections

rest. *See* relaxation; sleep

rheumatism, 82

S

sciatica, 213–17

self-acceptance, 42–43, 146, 150; Hawthorn Rose Honey, 149; Sweet Acceptance Tincture, 118

self-care, 1–2, 3, 13, 33–43; accountability for, 39; boundaries as, 36; in difficult times, 97; emotionality as, 40–41; hydration as, 34, 164, 207; individualized, 18, 19–22, 21, 23–24; movement as, 40; pleasure as, 37–38; principles from traditional wisdom, 18; rest as, 37, 121; ritual as, 124; seasonality of, 27–28, 30–31; self-acceptance as, 42–43; social movements and, 4–5; support as, 35, 186–88; vitality and, 79, 80

sex, 40, 84, 99, 159, 184, 186

shame, 11, 41, 108, 143, 153, 159, 184; food and, 60, 61; Heart Renewal Tincture, 148

shingles, 86, 216; Nerve Nourish Body Oil, 217

sinuses. *See* respiratory system

About the Author

BRITTANY DUCHAM is a community herbalist and writer bridging plant, personal, and political. She currently resides in Western Pennsylvania with her pup, Josie. Brittany carries a passion for bioregional herbalism, social justice, and DIY culture into her work, self-publishing zines and making small-batch herbal medicines. She runs Spellbound Herbals and Sensual Delight Press and her work can be found in herbal apothecaries and shops across the country.

Roost Books
An imprint of Shambhala Publications, Inc.
4720 Walnut Street
Boulder, Colorado 80301
roostbooks.com

Cover and interior art: Elana Gabrielle
Cover design: Kara Plikaitis
Interior design: Lizzie Allen
Typesetting: Kate Huber-Parker

9 8 7 6 5 4 3 2 1

First Edition
Printed in the United States of America

The information presented here is thorough
and accurate to the best of our knowledge.
Please do not attempt self-treatment of
a medical problem or condition without
consulting a qualified health practitioner.
Shambhala Publications and the author
disclaim any and all liability in connection
to the use of the instructions in this book.

⊛ This edition is printed on acid-free
paper that meets the American National
Standards Institute Z39.48 Standard.
♻ This book is printed on 30%
postconsumer recycled paper.
For more information please visit
www.shambhala.com.
Roost Books is distributed worldwide
by Penguin Random House, Inc., and
its subsidiaries.

Library of Congress
Cataloging-in-Publication Data
Names: Ducham, Brittany, author.
Title: Radical remedies: an herbalist's guide
to empowered self-care / Brittany Ducham.
Description: First edition. | Boulder,
Colorado: Roost Books | Includes
bibliographical references and index.
Identifiers: LCCN 2020013820 |
ISBN 9781611806724 (trade paperback)
Subjects: LCSH: Materia medica,
Vegetable—Popular works. | Herbs—
Therapeutic use—Popular works. |
Self-care, Health—Popular works.
Classification: LCC RS164 .D78 2021 |
DDC 615.3/21—dc23
LC record available at https://lccn.loc.
gov/2020013820